Understanding
Breast Cancer

Understanding Illness and Health

Many health problems and worries are strongly influenced by our thoughts and feelings. These exciting new books, written by experts in the psychology of health, are essential reading for sufferers, their families and friends.

Each book presents objective, easily understood information and advice about what the problem is, the treatments available and, most importantly, how your state of mind can help or hinder the way you cope. You will discover how to have a positive, hopeful outlook, which will help you choose the most effective treatment for you and your particular lifestyle, with confidence.

The series is edited by JANE OGDEN, Reader in Health Psychology, Guy's, King's and St Thomas' School of Medicine, King's College London, UK.

Titles in the series

KAREN BALLARD Understanding Menopause

SIMON DARNLEY & BARBARA MILLAR Understanding Irritable Bowel Syndrome

LINDA PAPADOPOULOS & CARL WALKER Understanding Skin Problems

PENNY TITMAN Understanding Childhood Eczema

MARIE CLARK Understanding Diabetes

MARK FORSHAW Understanding Headaches and Migraines

JOY OGDEN Understanding Breast Cancer

Understanding Breast Cancer

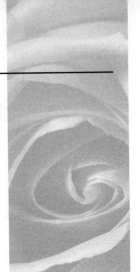

JOY OGDEN

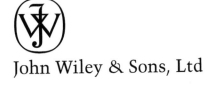

John Wiley & Sons, Ltd

Other Wiley Editorial Offices

John Wiley & Sons Inc., 111 River Street, Hoboken, NJ 07030, USA

Jossey-Bass, 989 Market Street, San Francisco, CA 94103-1741, USA

Wiley-VCH Verlag GmbH, Boschstr. 12, D-69469 Weinheim, Germany

John Wiley & Sons Australia Ltd, 33 Park Road, Milton, Queensland 4064, Australia

John Wiley & Sons (Asia) Pte Ltd, 2 Clementi Loop #02-01, Jin Xing Distripark, Singapore 129809

John Wiley & Sons Canada Ltd, 22 Worcester Road, Etobicoke, Ontario, Canada M9W 1L1

Wiley also publishes its books in a variety of electronic formats. Some content that appears
in print may not be available in electronic books.

Library of Congress Cataloging-in-Publication Data

Ogden, Joy
    Understanding breast cancer / Joy Ogden.
        p.   cm.
    Includes bibliographical references and index.
    ISBN 0-470-85435-9   (pbk.   :   alk.   paper) – ISBN 0-470-85435-9
    1.   Breast – Cancer – Popular works.   I.   Title.
RC280 .B80355 2004
616.99'44906–dc22
                                                2003027617

British Library Cataloguing in Publication Data

A catalogue record for this book is available from the British Library

ISBN 0-470-85435-9

Illustrations by Jason Broadbent

Typeset in 9.5/13pt Photina by Laserwords Private Limited, Chennai, India
Printed and bound in Great Britain by TJ International, Padstow, Cornwall
This book is printed on acid-free paper responsibly manufactured from sustainable forestry
in which at least two trees are planted for each one used for paper production.

Contents

About the author

JOY OGDEN is an award-winning health journalist of nearly 20 years' standing, who has written for a range of professional health titles such as *Nursing Times, Nursing Standard, Health Service Journal* and *Therapy Weekly*. She has contributed to national newspapers such as *The Guardian, The Observer, The Independent* and magazines such as *Yours Health Plus*. She is managing editor of *Acupuncture in Medicine*. Joy has recently had treatment for breast cancer and draws on her own experiences of living with its effects and her re-acquaintance with the NHS as a patient.

Acknowledgements

I would like to thank all the people who talked to me about their experiences of living with breast cancer. Their comments and contributions were generous, full of insight and extremely valuable – both for this book and for my own understanding, as someone who also lives with breast cancer.

I would like to thank my family and friends – and especially my two wonderful daughters, Louise Jones and Jane Ogden – for their unstinting and invaluable support and encouragement when I was coming to terms with my own diagnosis. Thanks to Jane also, as editor of this series, for her support in writing this book, and to Dr Polly James for her useful advice.

Introduction

As a health journalist I thought I knew a lot about cancer and my own chances of getting it. Looking around my long-lived, relatively cancer-free family I blithely assumed I was safe. It's true that my father died of lung cancer at the age of 59, but that was after a lifetime – starting at 13 – of chain-smoking. Oh, and his sister died of cancer, but she was also a very heavy smoker, so I never felt that counted either. I concentrated, instead, on the fact that all four of my grandparents lived well into their 80s or 90s, and that my mother is a miracle of fitness who survived a major car crash on a bridge holiday in France a couple of years ago at the age of 87 without a broken bone.

Well, I was wrong. I was sitting in the bath one Saturday night in March 2002 when I felt a shooting pain in my right breast. It felt – in retrospect at least – as though I was following a neon arrow pointing to The Lump. At first I thought I must be mistaken. But no, it did seem like a definite lump. That night I slept fitfully and every time I woke I reached again to feel for it, hoping that perhaps I had been mistaken. It was an agonising wait until Monday morning, when I went to the GP as an emergency appointment.

He was very kind. A bad sign, I thought. 'It doesn't feel like a bad lump,' he said. But nevertheless he said he would fax the consultant at the local hospital and I should get an appointment within two weeks. Two weeks. Two weeks sipping cold white wine by a pool in the south of France is no time at all. This was two weeks sitting in the dentist's chair with the drill whirring in my mouth. At the end of the first week I was an emotional wreck and rang the hospital to see when I could see the consultant. A pleasant-sounding receptionist assured me they had the letter and if it was considered urgent I would be seen as soon as possible. I just started quietly weeping, unable to control myself and unable to answer. I put the phone down. Half an hour later she rang and said they realised how distressed I was and the consultant would see me the following day. So that's how the long journey began. My cancer was malignant, but thankfully very small and there was no trace of it in the lymph nodes. I had a lumpectomy, followed by radiotherapy. The receptionist's kindness and understanding was typical of the treatment I received from everyone in the following weeks. I'm a seasoned complainer about poor service, but you won't hear me knock the NHS or the people who work in it.

I coped with my own diagnosis by reading everything I could find, trawling through the internet for information, and by talking to my family and friends. This book contains both facts and figures and the perspective of people who have experienced the different diagnoses and forms of treatment. This book aims to provide the sort of information and support that I was looking for. I hope that it will be a useful resource for others who have been diagnosed with breast cancer, as well as for their family and friends and for health professionals who come into contact with them.

What is breast cancer?

Overview

This chapter will look first at cancers in general and then in more detail at breast cancer. To give a clearer understanding of the different types of breast cancer, there is a brief description of the structure of the breast. There are explanations of the different types of tumours – non-invasive and invasive – and of secondary breast cancer.

What is cancer?

There is no one disease called 'cancer' which will one day be curable with a single remedy. It is a group of many different diseases that have some important things in common.

Cancers all develop as the result of cells which have run out of control and they all begin in the same way in the body's basic building block of life – the cell. The body has billions of cells of many different types which are grouped together to form tissues and organs. Normal cells grow in a controlled way and are constantly dividing to repair damaged tissues, to replace old cells and for tissues to grow. This helps to keep our body healthy. But normal cells only divide or reproduce when there is a need. Cells in tissues such as the skin or blood, for instance, are constantly wearing out and being replaced. When we cut ourselves, the cells around the injury will reproduce in order to repair and replace the damaged tissue, but once they have repaired it and the wound is healed they stop dividing. Sometimes, however, the control system goes wrong: the 'switch-off' mechanism fails and the cells become abnormal. Instead of stopping, the abnormal cells just keep on multiplying and dividing until a lump forms. This lump of extra tissue is called a tumour. It is thought that most invasive breast cancers have been present from 6 to 10 years before they are picked up by a mammogram or felt as a lump.

Are all tumours cancerous?

Not all tumours are cancerous, some are non-malignant or benign; that is, as it sounds, harmless – except when they grow in places where the pressure they exert causes a problem (for example large benign brain tumours). They are made up of cells that are quite like normal ones – and don't usually need to be treated. Benign tumours tend to grow very slowly, if at all, and don't spread beyond the tissue where they first started and into the rest of the body.

Malignant tumours, though, are made up of cancer cells that look abnormal and are not like the cells from which they developed. As a rule, the more abnormal (or anaplastic) the cells look, the more aggressively the cancer grows. Malignant tumours continue growing into surrounding areas and can spread to other parts of the body. It's this ability to damage and destroy surrounding tissues and to travel to other organs, where they grow as secondary (or metastatic) tumours, which makes cancerous cells so dangerous.

A malignant tumour which can invade and damage nearby tissues and organs is cancer. A benign tumour which will not spread to other parts of the body is not cancer.

What is meant by 'primary cancer'?

The place where a cancer starts is called the 'primary cancer'. Tumours from cancers that have spread are called 'secondary cancers' (doctors call these 'metastases' and they say a cancer that has migrated from its original site has 'metastasised').

So what is breast cancer?

Breast cancer, too, is not just one disease, but several. It can be found in a pre-cancerous state (which might go on to develop into invasive cancer if it is not treated), as a cancer which has not yet spread, or after it has spread to other organs. It can grow very fast or very slowly or somewhere in between. Breast lumps are common in women of all ages, but in younger women, particularly, they are usually non-malignant. Though it is rare, men can and do also get breast cancer.

Breasts are composed mainly of fat and breast tissue, together with nerves, veins, arteries and the connective tissue that helps to keep it all in place. The main

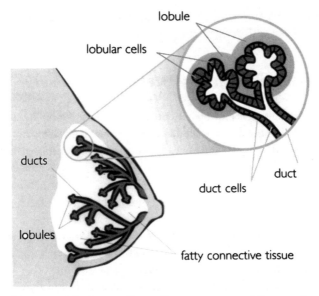

Figure 1. Diagram of the breast. From *Breast cancer: spot the symptoms early.* Leaflet by Cancer Research UK (2002). Reproduced by permission.

chest muscle is behind the breast and in front of the ribs in the chest wall. The breast (see Figure 1) is divided into around 20 lobes which look something like bunches of grapes. The 'grapes' are called lobules and the 'stems' are called ducts. The lobules produce milk and the ducts, which are thin tubes, transport the milk from the lobules to the nipple openings during breastfeeding.

Strands of fibrous tissue and globules of fat develop around the lobules and ducts in the breast during puberty. The breast also contains vessels carrying blood and lymph. Lymph is a yellow fluid that bathes cells. It is derived from blood as it passes through the blood vessels within a tissue, and is returned to the blood after passing through lymph glands. It flows through the lymphatic system throughout the body to help fight disease. The lymph vessels lead to lymph nodes, small bean-shaped organs which can trap bacteria or cancer cells travelling through the body in the lymph. There are clusters of lymph nodes near the breast in the axilla (under the arm), above the collarbone and in the chest. Benign or malignant tumours can develop in any of the breast's tissues – skin, gland, duct, fat, nerves, muscles, blood vessels or fibrous tissue.

Male breast tissue normally remains undeveloped, with rudimentary ducts ending in tiny lobular buds, like that of females before puberty.

After the menopause, when the ovaries stop producing hormones, the number of lobules decreases, and those that are left shrink. This means that the breasts, which are then composed of a higher proportion of soft fat, are less dense. And this means that interpretation of the X-rays is more reliable, so mammography is more likely to be effective in picking up abnormalities in post-menopausal women than in younger women with denser, firmer breasts.

What are the different types of breast cancer?

There are two main types of breast cancer – non-invasive or 'in situ' (cancers that are confined to the ducts or lobules and have not spread beyond the layer of tissue where they developed) and invasive (cancers that have started to spread into surrounding tissue).

Non-invasive ('in situ')

Ductal carcinoma (cancer) in situ (DCIS) is non-invasive and is becoming more common because it is picked up at an early stage on mammograms. If there is DCIS it means there are cells in the milk ducts of the breast that have started to grow and divide abnormally and turn into cancer cells. But they have not yet broken out of the ducts and developed the ability to spread either to the rest of the breast or the rest of the body. There is a very high chance that the cancer will be cured and will not recur if it is removed at this stage.

Some doctors call this a very early form of breast cancer, but others describe it as a pre-cancerous condition because it might develop into a more serious invasive cancer if it isn't treated.

Lobular carcinoma in situ (LCIS) means there are abnormal cells in the lining of the milk lobule. This is not considered to be breast cancer at this stage, but it does mean there is more risk of getting invasive breast cancer in either breast in the future. It is more common in women who are pre-menopausal and should be closely monitored.

Invasive

Ductal carcinoma is invasive and the most common type of breast cancer. It begins in the milk ducts of the breast but – unlike DCIS (see above) – it has developed the potential to spread to other parts of the body. The cancerous cells could do this by invading either the lymph or blood vessels in the breast and then being carried through them to other parts of the body, where they form other tumours. Because they have the potential to spread doesn't necessarily mean they have done, but doctors will want to assess the likely risk of it having happened, and if so how extensively, before deciding what treatment to recommend. This assessment is called 'staging'. (See Chapter 7 for definitions of cancer stages.)

Lobular carcinoma is an invasive cancer that begins in the lobules where milk is produced. It does not always show up as a definite lump and so it can be difficult to diagnose, which means it might be larger than other types of breast cancer when it's diagnosed. It is also more common for it to be diagnosed in both breasts at the same time.

Inflammatory breast cancer is a rare type of advanced breast cancer. It happens when the cancer cells block the lymph channels in the breast, and these then become inflamed. Inflammatory breast cancer can be confused with a breast infection or an allergic reaction because the symptoms can come on quite suddenly and are very similar, making diagnosis difficult. The first symptoms are usually a redness and warmth in the skin of the breast, often without a distinct lump. Other possible symptoms include sudden swelling – as much as a cup size in a couple of days – dark spots that look like bruises and a change in the colour of the areola (the dark area around the nipple). It can also show itself through ridges, welts, pitting and a change in colour – which can be difficult to see in women with darker skin tones. There might also be stabbing pains or persistent aches in the breast, discharge from the nipple and swollen lymph nodes under the arm or near the collarbone. If the breast is treated with antibiotics and fails to get better – or worse – it is important to have it investigated by a biopsy of the breast tissue and the skin itself. Inflammatory breast cancer grows and metastasises rapidly and must be taken very seriously.

Paget's disease is a rare invasive cancer which begins in the milk ducts of the nipple. One form of the disease is associated with an invasive cancer in the breast and another involves only the nipple. It often goes untreated until it is more advanced because its symptoms (including redness, oozing, crusting, itching of the nipple) are often thought to be due to an infection or inflammation. It is rarely found in both breasts, so if both nipples are itchy and scaling it is probably eczema, a far more common condition. If it doesn't clear up, however, it should be checked out. Paget's disease that involves the breast is treated as any other breast cancer, but when it involves only the nipple the cancer tends to grow slowly and can be treated by removing the nipple and areola.

Secondary breast cancer

The original cancer is the 'primary' cancer, so a secondary breast cancer is one that has developed from cancerous breast cells.

Tumours are made from millions of cancerous cells. Sometimes malignant cells that have grown into blood or lymph vessels break off and are carried round the body in the bloodstream or the lymph fluid. Once they have escaped they can become trapped in different organs, tissues, or lymph nodes, where they form a new tumour. Sometimes breast cancer cells that have migrated die and sometimes they lie dormant for many years. No one knows why some remain inactive or why some are reactivated years later.

Cancer can reappear either locally (close to the primary cancer site) or somewhere else in the body. If it recurs locally – in the skin over where the lump used to be, the scar from a mastectomy or in the remaining breast tissue after a lumpectomy – it is often because a few cancer cells were left there and have grown into a new tumour, and not because they have spread through the blood or lymphatic system.

Secondary breast cancer is more likely to occur in some parts of the body than others, commonly in: the lymph nodes near the breast (especially in the armpit, or the lower neck or chest); one or more bones; the lungs; the liver; and, sometimes, the brain. It is possible for it to affect more than one area at a time, but often it only affects one part of the body.

The earlier any recurrence is found and treated, the better is the outlook for the patient.

Summary

- Cancer cells lose the mechanism for dividing and self-destructing in an orderly way, become abnormal and continue to divide when new cells are not needed, thus producing a tumour.

- The place where a cancer starts is called the 'primary cancer'.

- A malignant tumour is one that can invade and damage nearby tissues and organs.

- A benign tumour will not spread to other parts of the body and is not cancer.

- There are two main types of breast cancer: non-invasive, that has not yet developed the ability to spread either to the rest of the breast or to the rest of the body; and invasive, that has the potential to spread to other parts of the body.

- Tumours that have spread to other parts of the body are called 'secondary cancers' or 'metastases'.

Who gets it? What are the risk factors?

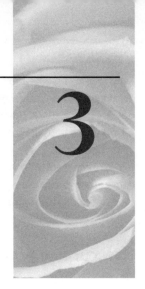

3

Overview

No one can pinpoint any one cause of breast cancer, but studies suggest some clues about the things that increase the chances of developing it. This chapter will set out some of the statistics and look at some of the more well-established risk factors together with some others which have been suggested and are being investigated. It examines in more detail the risks associated with HRT and in relation to ethnicity. It also looks at the risks of developing breast cancer 'because it runs in the family' and the issue of genetic testing.

How common is breast cancer?

Breast cancer appears to have reached epidemic levels. Talk to any group of people anywhere in the UK and they all seem to have some experience of it – someone in their family, a friend, a neighbour or work colleague. And it is not just a vague impression that this is the case, there are hard statistics to back it up. Every year around 39 000 women and between 200 and 300 men are diagnosed with breast cancer in the UK. Government figures show that the number of people who develop breast cancer every year has increased by 70 per cent since 1971, and by 15 per cent in the ten years to 2000. It is by far the most common form of cancer in women and the most common cause of cancer death in women.

The stark fact is that one in nine women will develop breast cancer at some time in their lives. Around 80 per cent of them will be post-menopausal when it happens – most commonly aged between 60 and 64. Contrary to widespread belief, age is undoubtedly the biggest risk factor, and the odds of developing breast cancer keep rising as women get older. Only 5 per cent of breast cancers (around 2000) are diagnosed in women under the age of 40, and 2 per cent (800) in women under 35. And while 13 000 women might die from the disease in any one year, almost all will have been diagnosed some years before. In a great number of cases, many years before.

Women from more affluent backgrounds are at higher risk of developing breast cancer than those from poorer environments. And people who live in the south of England and Wales are at more risk than those in the north of the UK.

How curable is breast cancer?

The latest survival figures for England and Wales show that while the numbers who get breast cancer are going up, the numbers who die from it are falling: almost three-quarters of women diagnosed with breast cancer in 1991–95 were alive five years later, and that rises to 78 per cent for women diagnosed in 1996–99. Five-year survival rates increase to 92.5 per cent where the cancer is detected by screening. The number of young and middle-aged women dying from breast cancer has been cut by almost a third since 1980 and three out of four women can now expect to beat the disease. Tamoxifen, the widely prescribed anti-oestrogen drug that has been used for more than 20 years, both to slow or stop tumour growth and to prevent recurrence, has contributed to the improvement in survival rate. The recently launched alternative, anastrozole (brand name, Arimidex), performs a similar function, but appears to be even more effective and to have fewer side effects. Breast cancer is the focus of a great deal of research around the world and new, improved diagnostic techniques, drugs and treatment are constantly improving survival rates. (See Chapter 12 for more information about tamoxifen and anastrozole.)

How will I know how likely it is that I'll be cured?

No one can be completely sure about the outcome of treatment, but there are a number of indicators. Breast cancer specialists in Nottingham have worked out a formula (the Nottingham Prognostic Index, or NPI) for the likely chances of a cure. It is based on three factors: the tumour size; whether or not it has spread to the lymph nodes and if so, how many; also the cancer's grade, which indicates how aggressive it is. It is a useful guide but it is only that, either in favourable or unfavourable predictions of outcomes. The formula is:

$$\text{NPI} = (0.2 \times \text{tumour diameter in cms}) + \text{lymph node stage} + \text{tumour grade}$$

Lymph node stages are: 1 (no nodes affected); 2 (1 to 3 nodes affected); 3 (4 or more nodes affected).

Tumour grades are: 1 (less aggressive); 2 (moderately aggressive); 3 (more aggressive) [see Chapter 7].

The formula produces scores in three bands:

- less than 3.4 suggests a high chance of cure
- between 3.4 and 5.4 suggests a moderate chance of cure
- more than 5.4 suggests a smaller chance of cure

But the NPI is only a guide and not infallible.

Male breast cancer

Men can and do get breast cancer, but it is rare and accounts for less than 1 per cent of all breast cancers. Between 200 and 300 men are diagnosed each year in the UK, and there are an estimated 3000 men across the UK who have the condition.

As with women, men are liable to get different types of breast cancer and, as with women, the commonest type is invasive ductal carcinoma. Pre-invasive ductal carcinoma in situ and inflammatory breast cancer are especially uncommon in men.

What causes breast cancer?

No one fully understands why people develop breast cancer but it seems certain that it has many causes that interact with each other in ways we don't yet understand.

Doctors and researchers agree that knocks and bruises do not cause the cancer, despite the fears that some people express. The things they have identified as risk factors fall into two categories – some fairly well supported by evidence and some still being researched. Some of these factors can be controlled – such as diet, weight, exercise, alcohol consumption – while others, such as family history and age are beyond our control. But knowing that there is a high risk can raise levels of awareness and vigilance, so that the cancer is picked up an early stage when the likelihood of curing it is greater.

Breast cancer is more common in women whose breasts have been subjected to oestrogen for longer. A woman who started her periods before the age of 12 is about one and a half times more likely to develop breast cancer than someone who started later. A woman whose periods end after the age of 55 is slightly more at risk, as is a woman who has her first child after the age of 30 or one who chooses to bottle-feed her babies. There is also evidence that women who take the Pill and HRT have a slightly higher risk of developing breast cancer.

Some research has identified the following as risk factors:

- Increasing age is by far the greatest risk – about half of breast cancers are in women aged between 50 and 64, and a further 30 per cent are in women over 70.

- Lengthy exposure to oestrogen, through
  - early start to menstruation (before age 12)
  - late start to menopause (after 55)
  - late age at first birth (age 30-plus)
  - never having children
  - being overweight after the menopause.

- Family history – only about 5–10 per cent of breast cancer cases are caused by an inherited faulty gene, but the more close relatives with breast cancer – especially at a young age – the higher the risk.

- Previous history of breast cancer. Women who have had breast cancer have a higher risk of getting it again in the same breast or a new cancer in the other one.

- Previously diagnosed benign breast disease.

- Radiation therapy – women whose breasts were treated with radiation therapy before age 30 are at increased risk.

Some studies indicate the following could also increase the risks:

- Taking hormone replacement therapy (HRT) for more than five years. Taking a combination of oestrogen and progestogen (synthetic progesterone) seems to carry a greater risk than with oestrogen alone.

- Birth control pill – slight increased risk in women while they are taking it, but this disappears 10 years after they stop taking it. The research, however, relates to older types of pill that had more oestrogen and progesterone and could have had a different effect on breast cancer risk.

- Alcohol – some convincing evidence that as consumption rises so does the risk, regardless of the type of drink – beer, wine or spirits.

- High fat diet – some suggestion that this is a risk factor, but not proven.

- Stress and anxiety – according to a recent Swedish study, but needs further research to be confirmed.

- Pesticides – some studies suggest that organochlorine pesticides, such as DDT, which are known oestrogenic compounds, could increase risks of breast cancer.

- IVF treatment for infertility – no proof yet, but widespread suspicion that it increases the risk.

Despite the many theories and the few established risk factors, doctors are still unable to pinpoint why any one woman develops breast cancer. Many women who do so have none of these risk factors, except for the risk that comes with growing older. And many women with known risk factors do not get breast cancer.

Some of these risk factors will now be covered in more detail.

HRT and breast cancer

Throughout the last decade hormone replacement therapy (HRT) has been pre-scribed for increasing numbers of women in their 50s and 60s to alleviate menopausal symptoms. Now it is coming under scrutiny as a possible factor in breast cancer. Researchers in America stopped part of a major study of combina-tion HRT (oestrogen–progestogen) three years earlier than planned, when initial findings showed that women on the drug had a higher risk of breast cancer, heart disease, stroke and blood clots. The findings indicated that the risk of breast cancer almost doubled for women after taking the combined oestrogens and progestogens (the artificial form of the female hormone progesterone) for more than five years. Actual numbers are still small, however, with an increase from 20 per 1000 women to 39, and many studies indicate that fewer women who develop breast cancer while using HRT actually die from the disease. The risk of developing breast cancer appears to be much less for women who take oestrogen-only HRT; however, this is shown to increase the risk of endometrial cancer.

There is still some dispute about how convincing the evidence is that HRT causes breast cancer, but it is more generally agreed that combined HRT use increases breast density, making it more difficult to interpret mammography, and therefore reducing the effectiveness of breast screening.

Breast cancer and ethnicity

Some cancers are more common in some ethnic groups than others, but it is difficult to unpick the influence of all the different variables in order to determine whether the most significant factor is genetic or environmental. Breast cancer is more common in women in the West: in Europe, North America, Australia and New Zealand and its incidence in these areas increased during the twentieth century. But it is not confined to the white women in Western countries. Asian or African women have a much lower incidence while they live in their traditional environment, but once they move to a Western country and adopt its lifestyle they also take on the higher incidence of breast cancer of their new neighbours.

Scientists have suggested that factors such as diet, the number of babies women have, the age at which they have them, and the length of time they breastfeed them might all contribute to the different incidence of breast cancer in different populations.

How important are family history and genetics in getting breast cancer?

Recent discoveries about human DNA and constant coverage in the press have led to rising anxiety about inherited disorders and consequently to demand for medical advice on genetics. Many women believe that if their mother died from breast cancer they are at great risk. For the majority this is a mistaken belief because, although a family history of breast cancer does in some cases give women a higher risk of developing breast cancer, most will not; most of those who do will be aged over 50 when it happens.

In fact, abnormal genes are believed to account for between 5 and 10 out of every 100 breast cancers. Most of the genes implicated in breast cancer are tumour suppressors that have changed (or mutated) in such a way that they have lost their ability to suppress cell growth. The inherited genetic mutations leave cells free to grow in an uncontrolled way, and a tumour develops.

The two genes BRCA1 and BRCA2 are the most important of those associated with a higher risk of breast and ovarian cancers in families. About one in 1000 women has inherited a mutation in these genes. But, although the mutated gene puts women at greater risk, it is not certain that it will lead to cancer. It is not known whether it is an interaction with other genes, or something in the environment that triggers cancer. And if one parent has the faulty gene only half his or her children will inherit it. Those relatives without the faulty gene have the same risk of developing breast cancer as the rest of the population.

What is involved in genetic testing?

The gene testing process has to start by searching for mutations in the genes of a family member who has already had cancer. It is only after that person has agreed to give a sample for genetic testing that it is possible to have a meaningful search in their relatives' genes.

Where can you go to find out if you have a faulty gene?

Some hospitals set up family history units in the early 1980s to deal with genetic cancer risks, and in 2000 the government called for better assessment and counselling for those affected.

People with a family history of breast cancer might well be inclined to magnify their own risks, but if they are worried they should ask to talk to a nurse who is trained in counselling at a family history unit.

People who are referred to one of the units will be assessed for their likely risk of having an inherited faulty gene. This is done by drawing up a family health tree by asking detailed questions about things such as the number of their affected relatives, how closely they are related, their ages on diagnosis and the ratio of those affected to those unaffected in the family.

Women who are identified as medium or high risk will be taught about breast awareness and referred for regular mammography. Those considered to be high risk might want to decide whether to go through the genetics testing process, or possibly consider a prophylactic (preventative) mastectomy.

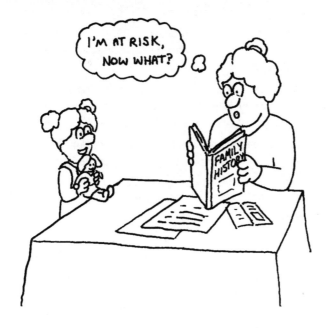

How do you decide whether to have a genetic test?

The decision about whether to have a genetic test or not should be made after careful consideration and discussion with health professionals who are experienced in dealing with the issue. Things to think about include:

- One reason to have the test is to be told you don't have the faulty gene. But if you are told you do, how will you cope?

- Women in their 20s, too young for mammography and not at high risk at that age, might find the knowledge that they have a risky breast cancer gene offers little chance to do anything about it and casts a shadow over their life.

- Having a genetic test might blight the chance of arranging a mortgage or insurance.

- The test might be useful if it motivates people to change their behaviour to reduce their risks – by attending for regular mammography, for example – but changing behaviour is often difficult.

Box 1.	Genes and breast cancer: some statistics.

- Faulty genes account for an estimated 2–5 per cent of all breast cancer.

- Although women who have a family history of breast cancer are at greater risk of developing the disease, most will not, and most who do will be over 50 when it happens.

- An estimated 8 per cent of women with one, 13 per cent of women with two, and 21 per cent of those with three affected close relatives go on to develop breast cancer.

- A high-risk breast cancer gene is more likely if there is a close relative who was aged under 50 when diagnosed, or there is more than one affected relative on the same side of the family.

- Cancer is common and cases can cluster in one family by chance, or because of low- or moderate-risk genes as yet unidentified.

- The genes BRCA1 and BRCA2 account for 1–2 per cent of all breast and ovarian cancers, but having the genes does not necessarily mean that either cancer will develop.

Some women (mistakenly) rush to the conclusion that they are at risk if their 65-year-old mother has breast cancer, while others with more reason for concern reassure themselves that it won't happen to them. The difference in attitude is illustrated by Caroline's story.

Caroline, who had a family history of breast cancer, put off going for mammograms, believing she would be safe:

“My mother had cancer of the ovaries, then breast cancer after that. She had just had her 59th birthday in hospital before she died, in 1992. And also my father's sister has had ovarian cancer, but she came through it. My doctor told me I should go for mammograms at 40 rather than 50 but I put it off for a year. I thought, Mum didn't get it till her early 50s and neither did my aunt, so I thought I'd be all right till the early 50s. I first went when I was 41 and they recommended I had mammograms every two years. But I found the lump myself, when I was 45, four months before I was due to go for a mammogram. I considered having this gene test done, then I chickened out because I thought, even if they tell me I have the gene they're not going to tell me what year I'll get it. I mean I could die of anything else before that. I could even get it in my 70s or 80s – and I'd go through all my life worrying, knowing that I'd got the gene and I'm going to get it sometime. **"**

Caroline opted for 'the lot' – mastectomy and chemotherapy, to maximise her chances of eradicating the cancer. Her sister, who is 14 months older, is receiving genetic counselling.

Men and genetic testing

Mutated genes can be inherited by men as well as women, but the decision about genetic testing is likely to be clearer cut for men. Mammograms are not appropriate and a man obviously doesn't have the risk of ovarian cancer, so the knowledge that he is carrying a risky breast cancer gene is likely to be of little use to him, unless he has daughters and is concerned to alert them to the possible dangers.

John, an ex-army man, was 67 when he was diagnosed, and concerned that his cancer could have been caused by a faulty gene. He said:

"Deep down in my heart I thought this could be genetic and, if it is, it's not fair on the children. I was very relieved when he came back and said I was clear. Seven years before I found the lump in my breast I'd lost my wife to cancer (of the jaw) and my mother had died of breast cancer at 54. I've done the genetic test, because obviously my daughter was quite concerned that both her grandmothers and her mother had died from different cancers. I've had the results and they say that 'within the current methods of testing' I do not have the genes, which is a big relief for my daughter. That's why I had it done. **"**

Summary

- About 39 000 women and 200–300 men are diagnosed with breast cancer every year in the UK but the number of young and middle-aged women dying from the disease has fallen by almost a third since 1980.

- No one knows the cause of breast cancer, but age is by far the greatest risk, with 80 per cent of cases occurring in women aged over 50.

- Another well-established risk factor is lengthy exposure to oestrogen through early start to menstruation, late onset of menopause or late age at birth of first child.

- Other suggested risk factors include taking HRT for more than 5 years, high animal fat diet, obesity in post-menopausal women and alcohol consumption.

- Breast cancer is more common in women in the West, but when Asian or African women adopt a Western lifestyle their risks are very similar to those of women in their new environment.

- Faulty genes account for only about 5 per cent of all breast cancer.

- The two genes BRCA1 and BRCA2 are the most important so far identified of those associated with a higher risk of breast and ovarian cancers in families.

Symptoms and diagnosis

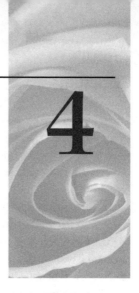

Overview

It is important that women are aware of how their breasts feel normally, so they will notice any change at an early stage, when treatment often has a better outcome. This chapter sets out the NHS's advice on breast awareness, outlines some of the most common types of non-malignant lumps and describes the symptoms of breast cancer. It details the ways in which doctors make a diagnosis and explains the signs that indicate the cancer has spread.

Breast awareness

The NHS Cancer Screening Programmes recommend that women should become aware of how their breasts feel and look at different times of the month, because when they know what is normal for themselves they will be more likely to recognise any untoward changes. Men, too, should be on the alert for any changes in their breast tissue. There is no evidence that a formally taught self-examination at the same time each month is more effective than a more relaxed attitude, they say, but they give the following five-point plan for breast awareness:

- Know what is normal for you.
- Look and feel.
- Know what changes to look for.
- Report any changes to your doctor without delay.
- Attend for breast screening if aged 50 or over.

Symptoms

Breast cancer can be present for years without causing any symptoms. The first sign that something is wrong for most women is when they find a lump in the breast or the nearby armpit. Usually, in the early stages it is not painful, although sometimes there is some discomfort. When it is at a more advanced stage it is more likely to be painful, and might feel as though it is fixed to the overlying skin or underlying muscles. Sometimes the nipple develops a discharge or becomes inverted (because it is tethered to underlying tissues) or looks red or scaly.

Occasionally, no symptoms are noticed until the cancer has spread to another part of the body and the first evidence of trouble can be general symptoms, such as tiredness, loss of appetite and weight loss.

Many people mistakenly think they only need to be concerned by lumps, but any sudden change in the breast that lasts for more than a few days should be investigated. The wisest thing to do is to go to the GP and let her or him decide what needs to be done.

The following are possible symptoms and changes that need to be investigated:

- A lump or thickening in or near the breast.
- A lump or swelling under the arm.
- Changes in the size or shape of the breast, especially those caused by arm movements or by lifting the breasts.
- Dimpling or puckering of the skin of the breast.
- Changes in the look or feel of the skin of the breast, the nipple or the area around the nipple (e.g. warm, swollen, itchy, red or scaly).

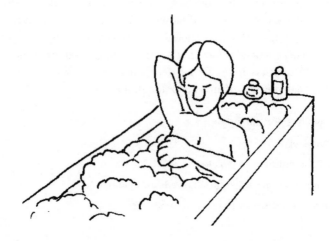

- Bleeding or discharge from the nipple.
- The nipple turns in and becomes inverted or points differently.
- Discomfort or pain in the breast, particularly if new and persistent.

Lumps

Breast lumps are very common in adult women of all ages, but especially in pre-menopausal women. Most women explore for lumps in the bath or shower, where wet, soapy fingers slide over the skin more easily. Eight out of ten lumps they find are benign – that is, not cancerous – and this is particularly true for younger women. These benign, non-malignant tumours are made up of cells that look the same, or almost the same, as the cells of the tissue from which they developed. They have clumped together into a lump but, unlike cancerous cells, they stop growing once they have reached a certain size.

A fibroadenoma is a smooth, rubbery or hard benign lump that is found most often in the breasts of teenagers or younger women. Solitary cysts (fluid-filled sacs) are among the most common benign breast lumps in women aged 35 to 55 and can be diagnosed and treated by needle aspiration of the contents of the cyst.

Although it is true that most breast changes are harmless, it is very important to get them all checked out by a doctor. Some women who are used to breasts with lumpy cysts take every new lump seriously, but others are so used to false alarms that they risk becoming complacent.

For instance Kay, who was aged 31 when she was diagnosed in 2001, says:

> ❝I was just in the bath, washing, when I came across the lump. I went to the doctor's after a couple of weeks and she said I should see a specialist. I didn't think it was anything – I thought it was a cyst because my Mum suffered badly from cysts when she was young. I went off on holiday while I was waiting for the appointment to come through. I had about two lumps on top of one another and another lump. I was extremely lucky it hadn't spread to the lymph nodes. I had to have a mastectomy – two days after my 32nd birthday – then chemotherapy and radiotherapy as well.❞

And Polly, a doctor training to be an anaesthetist, knew that at her age (31) the lump she found was probably nothing to worry about, so she left it a month before getting it checked out. She says:

> ❝I found just a small lump, which I wasn't really concerned about – I thought it was probably a little cyst or a fibroadenoma or something and I waited about a month to see whether it changed with my periods, which it

didn't do ... I wasn't feeling particularly worried by it at all. I took a little while, then went to see my GP who said she was sure it was nothing but she'd send me anyway to see the consultant. So I went to see him a few weeks later and he said he was sure it was nothing.**"**

But it turned out to be a grade three ductal carcinoma, for which she had a wide local excision, followed by chemotherapy then radiotherapy.

Women who are in the age groups most at risk of developing breast cancer (over the age of 45 or 50), or who have a strong family history of the disease, are advised to go for regular breast cancer screening.

Breast screening

Every woman in the UK who is registered with a GP will receive her first invitation to attend her local breast screening unit some time after her 50th birthday, and then every three years until her 65th birthday (see Figure 2).

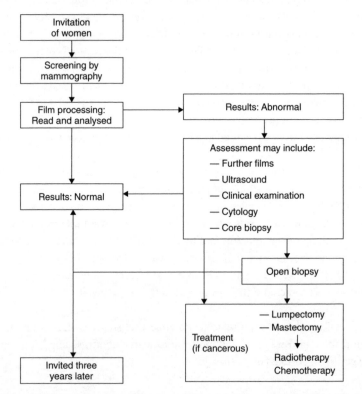

Figure 2. What happens at a breast screening unit? Image supplied, with permission, from the NHS Cancer Screening Programmes website, www.cancerscreening.nhs.uk.

There she will be asked if she has any symptoms or history of breast disease and will be given a mammogram, which is a low-dose X-ray. In a mammogram, each breast is placed on the X-ray machine and firmly compressed with a clear plate. It feels quite uncomfortable and some women say they find it slightly painful, but it only lasts a few seconds and does not harm the breasts.

The mammogram pictures are examined and the results are sent to the woman and her GP within two weeks.

The NHS says that about 95 per cent of women are given the all clear after the first mammogram and only about one in eight of those recalled for further investigation is found to have cancer.

Mammograms are a reliable way of detecting breast cancer early, but they are not foolproof. Some cancers are very difficult to see on the X-ray, some cannot be picked up on the X-ray at all, and sometimes the person reading it misses the cancer.

Jill's consultant did not rely on the mammogram for a diagnosis. Jill had gone to the doctor's about a minor problem and asked her to look at her right breast while she was there, because it looked a bit 'bunched up'. The doctor sent her for a mammogram:

> **❝**The mammogram didn't provide a conclusive picture because I was only 44 years old and had dense tissue in my rather enormous breasts. The consultant said he wasn't happy with it and extracted a cell sample with a needle. He asked me to return the very next day to have a proper biopsy where they cut out a little section of the dubious area to analyse it.**❞**

It turned out that Jill had lobular cancer.

How will the doctors make a diagnosis?

If the lump turns out to be suspicious, the GP will refer the patient to a surgeon in the breast clinic who will make the diagnosis after one or more of the following tests have been carried out:

- Palpation: the doctor – or sometimes a breast care nurse – can tell a lot about a lump just by feeling it and the tissue around it. They will examine both breasts with the flat of their fingers, also behind the nipple and under the armpit. A benign lump often feels different from a cancerous one to the doctor. A fibroadenoma is a smooth, round harmless lump that can be moved around easily and is very distinct from the rest of the breast tissue.

- Mammogram (low-dose X-ray): this involves compressing the breast and flattening it between two plates and can be quite uncomfortable, but it can give important information which will help in treatment and is over quite quickly. The mammogram is a less useful technique for diagnosing younger women because their breasts are denser – that is they have more active tissue and a lower percentage of fat than post-menopausal women – which makes it more difficult to read.

- Ultrasound: this uses high-frequency sound waves to scan the breast and is more useful than a mammogram in diagnosing younger women, whose breasts are denser. The doctor or radiographer who does the scan will apply gel to the breast then slide a blunt-ended probe over the surface and examine the image which appears on a screen. It is particularly useful in detecting breast cysts.

- Fine needle aspiration: a thin needle is used to remove material from a breast lump to discover whether it is a fluid-filled cyst or a solid mass (which might or might not be cancer).

- Core needle biopsy: a large needle can be used to remove a small cylinder of tissue from a lump that looks suspicious on a mammogram. It will be sent to a lab to be checked for cancer cells.

- Surgical biopsy: the surgeon cuts out part or all of a lump or suspicious area for examination.

Box 2.	Questions to ask following diagnosis.

- What stage is it? (See Chapter 7 for an explanation.)
- What kind of breast cancer is it?
- Is it invasive?
- What did the hormone receptor test show? (See Chapter 7 for an explanation.)
- What other tests were done on the tumour and what did they show?

People find their breast cancers in a variety of circumstances, for instance Molly, aged 62 when she was diagnosed in 1982, found hers at a routine smear test, when her doctor did a breast examination. She says:

> ❝He found the lump, which was quite small – right in the front of my breast just above the nipple. I got a very quick appointment at the hospital. The doctor thought it was benign so I wasn't too worried, and most lumps are.❞

Molly had a lumpectomy.

Because of its rarity, many men put off going to the doctor's when they first notice a change in their breasts. John, an ex-army man who was aged 67 when he was diagnosed in 2002, is married to a retired GP and she encouraged him to see his doctor. John says:

> ❝I was standing in the shower and thought, 'That shouldn't be there, I've got a lump in my breast.' I had a routine appointment with my GP the next day to have my blood checked. He gave me the talk which I would have expected any GP to give me, which was that lots of men get lumps, very rarely cancer. Within two days I saw (a specialist) who went through the same spiel and he had one of those machines which gave him a lovely picture of my chest. His first words were, 'Oh dear!' – and you think, 'Oh God! here you go.' He gave me a local anaesthetic and gave me a biopsy with a machine like a Flash Gordon ray gun. Within a few days they confirmed it was cancer and it was malignant ... I was booked in to have a hernia repaired three days later, so they took over the slot and in fact (the surgeon) did the mastectomy and the hernia at the same time.❞

Philip, who was 40 in March 2000 when he was diagnosed, was also encouraged by his partner to visit the doctor, and says that left to his own devices he might well have ignored it. He says:

> ❝I felt a slight pain in my breast and there was a little lump there. I went to see the doctor about a couple of weeks after. He thought it was just a cyst – he said, 'We'll monitor it, come back in a month.' It was still there after a month, so I went to see a consultant, who said, 'Don't worry it's only a cyst but we'll take it out anyway and do a biopsy.' He found out it was DCIS and said straight away, 'We want to give you a mastectomy,' which is what they did, and they took out 19 lymph nodes from under the arm. Luckily they were free and that was very good. I had six months of chemo but no radiotherapy.❞

How do we know whether the cancer has spread?

There is no way of knowing with absolute certainty whether a cancer has spread, and the risk that breast cancer will spread is greater than for some other cancers. But the best indication about whether or not it has spread more widely is whether there are cancer cells in the lymph nodes in the armpit. (See Chapter 8 for more information.) The more lymph nodes that are found to have cancerous cells, the greater the risk that the cancer has already spread into the rest of the body – most commonly the bones, lungs or liver, though sometimes the brain.

The other warning sign is the degree of abnormality in the appearance of the cell. Cancer cells that look more like normal breast cells are less likely to spread than those that have become anaplastic and are difficult to recognise as breast cells at all.

When the cancer cells have spread to another part of the body – either in the bloodstream or the lymph fluid – they can become trapped in distant organs or tissues. There they sometimes die or remain inactive for years. But sometimes, for some unknown reason, they wake up and form a new tumour. The new tumour is called a secondary (or metastatic) cancer. Breast cancer cells which have spread to the lungs or liver are still breast cancer cells and the new tumour is secondary breast cancer, not lung cancer or liver cancer. The treatment for secondary breast cancer in the lungs is not the same as for lung cancer.

Secondary breast cancer

Local and regional recurrence

Sometimes microscopic cancer cells are left over from surgery and the cancer comes back in the same place as the original tumour or in the scar. This is called 'local' recurrence. If the cancer has come back in one of the lymph nodes under the arm or above the collarbone, it is called a 'regional' recurrence.

It is also possible to develop a new cancer in either breast, which might be many years after the original cancer and in a completely different area of the breast. If there is a new cancer in a breast which has been treated with radiotherapy the patient will need to have a mastectomy, as the breast cannot be treated in this way twice.

A local or regional recurrence does not necessarily mean that the cancer has spread beyond the breast to the rest of the body, but the first step in finding out if it has, is to do a series of tests. These include: bone scan to test for spread to the bone; X-ray to test for spread to the lungs or bones; ultrasound for examining liver and ovaries; CT scan (computerised tomography or body scan) to test for spread to the abdomen and liver; MRI (magnetic resonance imaging) to determine how extensive cancer is in the breast of a woman already diagnosed; and blood tests to check for spread to the liver and/or bones.

A secondary (or metastatic) breast cancer

Breast cancer that has spread to other organs is rarely cured. But this does not mean it cannot be treated. With the help of the medical profession, some women with secondaries can live for many years. The treatment given differs for each patient, depending on factors such as the aggressiveness of the original cancer, whether it was sensitive to hormones, how many places it has metastasised to and which organs are involved.

The general approach to treating patients with metastatic breast cancer is to maintain their quality of life, while lengthening their survival time. Hormonal therapy, immunotherapy and chemotherapy are the main treatments for metastatic cancer, with chemotherapy and radiotherapy to ease the symptoms.

It is important to discuss treatment with the doctors. Patients might feel that some treatments spoil their enjoyment of life without giving any improvement in their chances of remission, and so decide to stop treatment altogether. Palliative care, which controls the symptoms without treating the cause, can be given either at home or in a hospice, once that decision has been made.

What are the symptoms of secondary cancer?

Most women whose breast cancer has spread don't show any symptoms until the cancer has spread quite extensively.

The bones

The first sign for many is an ache in the bone, which makes it difficult to get to sleep and quite painful to move around. Sometimes it is difficult to tell if it is just low back pain or some other condition, like arthritis. But, unlike arthritis, where movement improves as the day goes on, bone pain caused by cancer is steady. Pain that lasts for more than a week or two should be checked out.

The liver

Breast cancer that has spread to the liver leaves the patient feeling unwell, more tired than usual, nauseous and with little appetite. It can also lead to a swollen abdomen and discomfort on the right-hand side of the abdomen. And the skin and whites of the eyes can become yellow and the skin itchy.

The lungs

People with secondary breast cancer in the lungs usually first notice when they become short of breath easily or have a chronic cough.

The brain

If a secondary breast cancer develops in the brain it can lead to headaches and nausea. Sometimes symptoms resemble those of a stroke – a weakness develops, there is unsteadiness in walking or you can't see out of one eye, depending on which part of the brain is blocked by the tumour.

Summary

- NHS Cancer Screening Programmes recommend that women should become aware of what is a normal state for their own breast, in order to recognise perverse changes.

- Breast cancer can be present for many months or years without causing symptoms, but changes that need to be referred to the doctor include lumps in the breast or armpit, changes in the size or shape of the breast, dimpling of the skin or changes in the nipple.

- All women should attend for three yearly breast screening after the age of 50.

- Final diagnosis follows a series of tests: mammogram, ultrasound, fine needle aspiration, core needle biopsy and/or surgical biopsy.

- There is no way of knowing for sure whether a cancer has already spread, but the best indicator so far is how abnormal the breast cells appear and whether or not it is present in the lymph nodes in the armpit.

Psychological impact – coming to terms with breast cancer

Overview

Women who are diagnosed with breast cancer have to come to terms with the trauma of a life-threatening illness and the possibility of mutilating surgery. This chapter looks at the ways in which people try to protect their psychological well-being through defence mechanisms such as denial or repression or by looking for meaning, searching for mastery and improving their self-esteem.

First reactions

It's one thing to hear dramatic announcements of life and death importance in soap operas on the television or in a play at the theatre, and quite another to experience them first-hand. The first reaction to the news that you have cancer is often one of disbelief. And immediately following on is the question – spoken out loud or just an unspoken but insistent shriek in the head – 'Am I going to die?' For a woman who is diagnosed with breast cancer the very next question is usually, 'Will I have to lose my breast?'

Most women, in fact, do not die of breast cancer and most do not lose their breasts but those are two of the main fears. Cancer has its own special place in the chamber of horrors. But breast cancer has its own special difficulties, too. Most women feel perfectly well when they go to the doctor's with a little lump and it's hard for them to believe that suddenly they have a life-threatening illness when they feel so fit and healthy. It's also hard to accept that the cure might mean accepting mutilation and the loss of something so intimately associated with their sexuality.

So how do women cope with the diagnosis of breast cancer? It's perhaps easier to view it as not one crisis, but a series of crises. First there is the shock of the diagnosis and adaptation to that; then the treatment, each stage of which (any combination of surgery, chemotherapy, radiotherapy, hormonal therapy and biological therapy [or immunotherapy]) presents another critical situation; then comes remission, which calls for further psychological adjustment.

The illness can cause major upheavals in the patient's life, including changes in the diversity of roles which contribute to their sense of unique identity (for instance, from chief parental family organiser to passive child-like patient); changes in their future expectations (for instance from a future with children to a childless one); as well as changes in the way their body looks and works. People who are not used to being ill and have not developed ways of coping are suddenly confronted with uncertainties about the seriousness of their condition and are under pressure to make important decisions about treatment. There is a lot of adjustment to be made and different people adopt different ways of protecting themselves from the psychological impact of a breast cancer diagnosis.

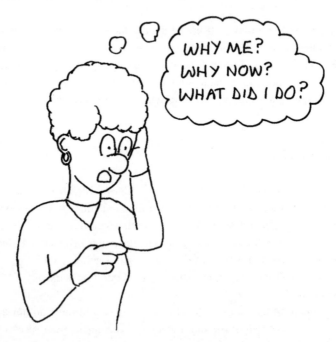

Typical defence mechanisms people use to protect themselves

Patients use a variety of psychological tactics to protect themselves from facing up to the change in present relationships and future expectations that a diagnosis of breast cancer entails. Here are a few of the more typical defence mechanisms they adopt:

- Denial – subconsciously denying the seriousness of the diagnosis (or ignoring a suspicious lump instead of going to the doctor); sometimes it is family and friends who deny the illness and play down anxieties or deliberately change the subject.

  Some of Molly's friends coped with her diagnosis by denying it:

  ❝[xx] is a great one for sticking his head in the sand, he won't face anything and [his wife] is a very confrontational slightly aggressive person, with a kind person inside trying to get out. They invited me to lunch every Sunday and one of them would give me a lift but they never talked about it, never asked how I was.**❞**

- Repression/suppression – more deliberately deciding not to think or talk about the cancer.

  One of Polly's friends, who refused point-blank to talk about the diagnosis, illustrates this response:

  ❝I told a friend, who said, 'Oh I can't talk about that, I'll have to phone you tomorrow when I've had time to think about it' – obviously very upset, but that's kind of weird.**❞**

- Displacement – transferring emotions or ideas from their original source to a more acceptable substitute (e.g. venting anger with the doctor or the illness on partner or children).

  Trish, who was worried by the prospect of radiotherapy, displaced her fears about its effect on her body to the staff who were delivering it:

  ❝The hospital staff were all very lovely, but it's a horrible thought all that radiation. I think I was quite rude and unpleasant to the staff for the first few times, looking back. And then gradually I felt I was taking charge of it.**❞**

- Projection – attributing unacceptable feelings to someone else (e.g. 'the doctor thinks I'm going to die').

  Gwen found herself projecting her own risky thoughts on to those around her, in an effort to deal with them:

  ❝You don't want to face up to the thought that you might die in the not-too-distant future, but that's precisely what cancer makes you do. It's easier, somehow, to put feelings like that at one remove and you find yourself shunting your fears off and attributing them to whoever's close at hand. **99**

- Rationalisation – finding plausible reasons to behave in a way that could be seen as intolerably risky (e.g. the cancer isn't so bad, so it won't make any difference if I stop chemo now).

    Gwen says she knows she is rationalising:

    66I can't bring myself to do all that self-examination thing – just in case I actually find something. Part of me says it's not a very efficient way of finding a lump – but that's how I found the lump in the first case for God's sake – so another part of my brain knows that's daft. **99**

- Reaction formation – repressing unacceptable feelings and expressing opposite ones (e.g. buying gifts as tokens of esteem for a consultant, who is perceived as arrogant and is disliked).
- Regression – slipping back into childlike ways of reacting.

    Polly, a doctor, was surprised at her own childlike response to the diagnosis:

    66One thing I knew when I was going through it was that I didn't want to make any decisions, which is surprising really … I just wanted someone to tell me what to do. Even the choice of, 'Do you want to do this clinical trial of this new chemotherapy?' … I just wanted to say, 'Well what do you think? What would you do if you were me?' Which kind of goes against all the modern NHS thinking. I was greatly relieved when anybody told me what to do because I really didn't want the responsibility of making the decision. **99**

- Sublimation – diverting unacceptable drives into personally and socially acceptable channels (e.g. channelling frustration at delays in screening into a campaign to improve services).

So how do people cope with breast cancer and adjust to it?

According to some psychologists, people respond to life-threatening events such as breast cancer in the following ways:

- Shock – disbelief and denial, feeling stunned and bewildered, behaving in an automatic way and feeling detached from the situation.
- Acute distress – feelings of loss, grief, anger, anxiety, helplessness and despair.

- Looking for meaning.
- Searching for mastery.
- Improving self-esteem.

This is not a template, however, and the meaning of the illness and the response depend on things such as:

- The disease itself – what stage it is in, whether it has spread, and whether the surgery and follow-up treatment will be radical or minimal.
- Stage of life – a young woman who might become infertile with chemotherapy is likely to find it much more devastating than a post-menopausal woman.
- Social support – access to the comfort and backing of family, friends or religion.
- The individual's own personality, inner resources, values and emotional patterns.

Shock, disbelief and denial – and acute distress

When breast cancer is diagnosed, before the search for meaning begins, the first response is often shock, numbness or disbelief. Cancer might be picked up in a seemingly healthy person at a routine mammogram, or it might have followed a failure to investigate earlier concerns. The initial emotional reaction is influenced by the way the diagnosis is made and the way it is announced, as well as by the patient's personality and attitudes. But whatever the circumstances surrounding the announcement, powerful emotions, such as fear, anxiety, depression, anger, panic and guilt, are frequently unleashed (though they are often disguised by outward acceptance and calm), and rapid mood swings are common.

Molly was 62 and recently retired from her job as a social worker when she was diagnosed. She was outwardly calm, but inwardly deeply shocked when she was told:

> **❝** The doctor thought it was benign, so I wasn't too worried. A friend insisted on coming with me – when you are single you get used to doing things by yourself and I wouldn't have bothered, but I was glad afterwards that she had ... the consultant said, 'Well, I think it's a growth.' He said it might mean removing my nipple, it might mean a mastectomy, which had always been a particular nightmare of mine ... My friend thought he had been a bit brutal. I was chatting away to her as though I'd had very good news and everything in the garden was beautiful, yet at the same time all this stuff was going on underneath. **❞**

Jill, who works in local government, was also in denial at the news that she had breast cancer:

> ❝It was just after Christmas and someone asked me out for lunch. I remember saying, 'Oh no I've got a hospital appointment on Tuesday, but Friday should be fine.' But Friday wasn't fine. By then the bottom had fallen out of my world. I may have got this wrong because the panic was buzzing round my head but I believe he explained that the type of cancer I had was 'lobular'. It spread behind the nipple and was a Stage 2 cancer about 3 cm long, so he recommended a full mastectomy followed by chemotherapy and radiotherapy and he prescribed tamoxifen straight away. I remember looking into his eyes with disbelief and saying, 'Are you sure?' as if the man didn't know his job – but I just kept thinking, this can't be happening to ME.❞

Polly, a registrar and training to be an anaesthetist, was 30 when she was diagnosed with a Grade 3 ductal carcinoma. Her medical training did not protect her from the shock and acute distress of the diagnosis. Because of her age, her GP and then her consultant assumed the small lump she had found was a harmless cyst and were as shocked as she was by the biopsy:

> ❝When I found out I think it was just total shock. I just felt ill all the time and couldn't do anything and felt like I didn't really believe it. But at the same time you felt that sort of sick thing when you know it's true. When he was telling me I just wanted to know exactly what was going on then get out of the door and go home. You don't want to hear – you don't even want to listen to it, or that's what I thought, I thought I just want to go now. I felt like I was being made to sit and listen to stuff I didn't want to hear.❞

Most people – at least in the Western world – don't really confront the fact that they will one day die. A diagnosis of cancer brings it home that they will. And it could be sooner rather than later. This has a profound impact on emotions. It brings a feeling of uncertainty about the future and of losing the ability to control any aspect of it.

Jill, aged 44 when she was diagnosed, had young children to care for and was desperate to survive for them as well as for herself:

> ❝I remember asking the surgeon about my chances and wishing I hadn't. He said, 'I have to think there is a 40 per cent chance of you surviving five years.' That was eight years ago – I'm obviously one of the lucky 40 per cent.❞

Looking for meaning (I know what caused my illness)

Throughout life we look for patterns to explain the world around us and to predict what will happen to us. A diagnosis of breast cancer exposes the flimsiness of our grip on the controls, so we search for an explanation of its cause and its implications for our life, in order to win back a feeling that we can shape what happens to us. Many women have their own explanation of why they developed the cancer – such as stress, HRT or a blow to the breast – sometimes with little basis in scientific evidence, but which nevertheless gives them a feeling that they know why it happened, and can therefore affect what happens to them in the future.

Katrina, who was in her early 40s when she found a lump, had no doubt in her own mind about its cause:

❝As soon as I felt the lump I thought, I know what this is about. That is why I have always seen it as an emotional issue rather than a physical cancer. Yes, I know what brought it on. When my children were very, very small my marriage ended. My husband got the children and I didn't see them for 10 years. I think the grief and the guilt I obviously felt, I couldn't deal with it. The depression was within me, I know it was. It wouldn't be in my left breast and so close to my heart.❞

Jill, aged 44 when she was diagnosed with lobular carcinoma, has her own views about what caused the cancer:

❝I reminded my surgeon that nine years previously I had come to him with a blocked milk duct after I'd been breastfeeding my son and that maybe that had something to do with it. He discounted this theory. We discussed the fact that both my mother and sister had died two years previously within 24 hours of each other. It may be that sometimes a traumatic shock can stop your body fending off the development of cancer cells which may lie dormant in all of us, acting as a type of catalyst for changes in the cell structure.❞

Afterwards, many also try to understand the long-term effects that having breast cancer has had on their lives. They often say that it has made them reappraise their life and given them a clearer idea of what should be given priority and what should be jettisoned as a waste of precious time. Through all this, the illness starts to have a meaning – 'things happen for a reason'.

Michele, who was diagnosed in October 2000, shortly after she had finished breastfeeding the youngest of her three children, found the news that she had a 50/50 chance of survival profoundly shocking, but is taking back control of her life:

❝It rocked my underlying confidence that everything will always be alright. I do feel more vulnerable. But in some ways it is a good thing – I look after myself better and it's really brought home the beauty of life and why it is so special to be here. I just feel very happy and lucky and thankful it has turned out well. It's just about having hope – being as realistic as you can, but daring to hope. There is so much you can do to help yourself, you don't have to be a victim of it all, however things turn out, if you take some control back.❞

A search for mastery (I can control my illness)

Many people approach treatment feeling relatively positive but become disheartened by the debilitating and upsetting side effects and changes to their bodies.

They try to find ways to control the illness, to stop it happening again and to give themselves a feeling of 'mastery' over their destiny. They do this through psychological techniques – such as developing a positive attitude, meditation or self-hypnosis, or by changing their behaviour in some way – adopting a different diet, changing medications, or searching for information on the internet.

Trish, 42 when she was diagnosed, found it difficult to accept the treatment that her doctors were recommending and went to the Bristol Cancer Help Centre to sort out her feelings and to help her regain a feeling of power over her future:

❝Within about ten days of finding the lump I had surgery – just a lumpectomy – it was early stage, the lymph nodes were clear and it was oestrogen positive ... They suggested I had chemotherapy and radiotherapy and they said – I remember it so clearly – 'You're young, you're fit, you've got a very good chance of surviving this.' I thought, 'Yes, I am young, I am fit and healthy and I don't really need all this' ... after Bristol I had radiotherapy but I didn't have chemo or tamoxifen. It wasn't what they told me at Bristol, it's what I felt I was able to cope with ... I went on a very strict vegan diet for about three years, then felt my body needed a bit more, so now I have oily fish once a month and also eat chicken livers once a month to help with my blood. I still eat organically and try and eat as much in season as I can. I always thought I ate quite well before, but on reflection I don't think I did. Now I don't touch dairy at all, and no tea, coffee, alcohol, sugar or salt.❞

Improving self-esteem (I'm better off than a lot of people)

Once the operation is over, there is sometimes a feeling of euphoria – perhaps because some of the uncertainty is relieved – also because of the prospect of returning to normal life.

Jill, who was 44 when she was diagnosed with lobular cancer that had spread to her lymph nodes, found that some of her fears were alleviated once the surgery was safely out of the way:

❝As I was wheeled into theatre I was still seeking reassurance from the nurse pushing my trolley that I had to have it done. Once the deed had been done, it was easier to cope with because there was no going back and it was far less painful than I expected. I had two drainage tubes and a bag attached to me which I carried about in a Tesco carrier bag when I wanted to go to the loo or chat to someone across the ward. It became like a girls' dormitory with us all sitting up in bed chatting and crying and laughing about our feelings and our lives. Eight years on, I'm still in touch with some of them.❞

But the euphoria is usually fleeting, and many women then experience a period of disbelief and denial, followed by anxiety. Their self-esteem has dwindled; they feel as though there is a constant threat hanging over them and are frightened by the smallest change in their bodies in case it means the cancer has returned. Most people eventually develop ways of coping, and many do this by making sense of their experience by comparing themselves (favourably) with others. Older women think they are better off than younger women, while younger women think they are better off than older women. Women who have had a lumpectomy thank their lucky stars they have not had a mastectomy, while women with a mastectomy thank heavens their cancer has not spread. The important thing, it seems, is not whether what you believe is true or not, but whether you can explain your illness to your own satisfaction and therefore adjust to it (see the 'Helpful tips' box with hints for the patient on how to cope).

Jill is coping with the change in her body and is wryly humorous about it:

❝I feel very lop-sided ... But as a fellow-sufferer once said, 'It's better to be lop-sided and alive than symmetrical and dead. And it'll improve your snooker skills enormously!'❞

Kay, who was 31 when she found the lump that was later diagnosed as cancer, is determined to get over the experience and get on with her life:

❝I did have moments of crying, but not a lot, very rare. To me it's been and done – it's not disrupted my life, there's a lot worse in life than losing a boob, so I just feel lucky and hope it won't go any further.❞

Molly:

❝I think it's interesting that after all these years (1979 when it all started) in talking about it, it's all as vivid as it ever was and perhaps it always is. But

I think there is a part of me that feels very good that I came through it all and that I recovered – because not everybody does. **"**

A minority find it difficult to adapt, and continue to suffer anxiety and depression or sexual problems for some years after surgery – and this seems to be as true for women who have had a lumpectomy as for those who have had a mastectomy.

Many women, however, find that being female – and being sexually attractive – is not just a matter of having two breasts. Many find a new meaning in their lives and view the cancer as a learning experience and a challenge to be overcome.

Trish has found the experience of breast cancer has affected her on an 'emotional, spiritual level far more deeply than a physical'. She said:

"I never thought I wouldn't get through it – I understood I wouldn't live for ever, but I didn't see it as that I might die – the biggest effect it had was that if I wanted to live my life the way I wanted to live my life I had to get this sorted. There were issues I had to address before I could start getting myself better. It was definitely a second chance.

I'd rather not have had cancer to be where I am now. But the only reason I am where I am now is because I have cancer. I think a lot of people feel that way. **"**

HELPFUL TIPS! HELPFUL TIPS! HELPFUL TIPS! HELPFUL

Hints for the patient on how to cope

- Coping is about dealing with the crisis of physical illness – but there is no right or wrong way of doing it, it's a question of finding what works for you.
- Take your medication and keep your doctor's appointments.
- Find out as much as you can in advance of treatment and examine the alternatives, to prepare yourself emotionally.
- If you wake up feeling depressed don't fight it – have a good cry and a good moan – then remind yourself that you'll probably feel better as the day goes on, so you can make breakfast, brush your teeth and gradually get on with life.
- Stay away from people and situations that make you feel stressed or depressed.

- Don't isolate yourself – having some time on your own is fine, but capitalise on the support of family and friends.
- Ease up on yourself – put off making major decisions and forget about being a perfectionist.
- Avoid alcohol – as well as being implicated as a risk factor in breast cancer, alcohol is a depressant, which is the last thing you want.
- Laughter is a good doctor – find a funny film or something that makes you smile.
- Keep a diary – expressing how you feel and keeping a record of it can be therapeutic.

Summary

- A diagnosis of breast cancer can cause major upheavals in the patient's life starting with shock, disbelief and denial, then acute distress, followed by gradual adjustment and acceptance.

- Patients typically adopt a variety of psychological tactics to protect themselves, such as denial, repression, displacement, projection and rationalisation.

- According to some psychologists people learn to cope with breast cancer by looking for meaning (I know what caused my illness), searching for mastery (I can control my illness), and improving self-esteem (I'm better off than a lot of people).

- The response to the illness, however, depends on things such as the stage of the disease, the patient's stage of life, access social support and the individual's own personality.

The role of family, friends and health professionals

6

Overview

This chapter explores ways that friends and relatives can help and looks at what to tell children. It also outlines ways that healthcare staff can support their patients.

How can friends and relatives help?

Friends and relatives can be a major source of support, but face their own difficulties. They have to provide emotional support, physical care and help in making decisions about treatment. Many of the observations about the impact of cancer are as true for them as for the patient. Their response to the illness depends on things such as their relationship to the patient, the stage of the disease and their own personalities.

Polly, aged 30 when she was diagnosed, feels her mother is finding it hard not to be over-protective. She said:

> **"**She just seems to want to go out and buy endless tablets from the health food shop, phones me up all the time, telling me to read things in *The Times* or something ... all of it is not appropriate or not what I want to do and she seems to be just wanting to put me to bed all the time – lots of rest and making sure I'm eating broccoli a lot ... It's difficult to be patient ... but I can understand why she wants me to.**"**

Some of Molly's friends were a great help, while others didn't quite know how to respond:

❝Some people would come up and give me a hug and say, 'How are you – having a bad time?' Those I found the best ones ... But one who really got under my skin – kindest possible person, she meant extremely well – used to come up to me and say, 'You're looking very well,' whatever I looked like, until one morning she said it to me once too often – I knew she darned well couldn't see me and I was feeling particularly grim and I rather turned on her. She said, some time afterwards, 'I thought that's what you wanted to hear.' Well, maybe some people do, but it didn't suit me because I knew it wasn't true.❞

Some men hide their distress about their partner's cancer, in the belief that this is the best way to support them. The women, on the other hand, often view this as insensitive and rejecting.

Jill's husband was intent on reassuring her, but she would have welcomed a more realistic attitude:

❝The worst thing for me was the false reassurance continually dealt out by my nearest and dearest. 'Don't be silly – you'll be alright' type of thing. We all know it's a condition that can kill and if I wanted to talk about making a will or the side effects I was experiencing, I needed to do just that.❞

Joan's husband is very supportive in practical ways, but finds it hard to talk about her cancer:

❝He really didn't want to talk about it – he won't talk about things that worry him. The only time he broke down was when we were talking to the breast care nurse. I asked her something and she went to find out and when she went out of the room he broke down. But apart from that he's brilliant – does all the ironing, most of the vacuuming.❞

Telling friends and loved ones is sometimes hard because their reactions mirror – and reinforce – the patient's own. Some people feel guilty and want to protect those they love from these emotions, and some worry that the news that they have cancer will create a distance between them and their loved ones. But by sharing the diagnosis, people can share their feelings and offer each other love and support.

Polly, aged 30 when she was diagnosed in February 2003, dreaded telling her family, but found their support made all the difference:

❝Generally when I first found out, I couldn't bear to tell anybody. I remember phoning up my sister – the first person I told – and I thought, 'Oh, it's going to be awful and I'm ruining her week by telling her this.' And she was very, very pragmatic about it and immediately said, 'That's terrible – but – you're going to have a horrible year but you're just going to do it and get through it.' And that was very good actually. **99**

Molly, too, found it hard to tell those closest to her, but as time has moved on she has been more able to share her feelings:

66I suppose my sister was the one most adversely affected ... She has a long history of clinical depression ... I'd always felt that I needed to protect her a bit, and partly because I was so busy coping for myself – and partly because I didn't really want to – I didn't talk to her. I thought I was protecting her, but she felt very cut off and she found a counsellor. She told me that her biggest fear was the rift between us would be for ever, that she'd 'lost me' and if it hadn't been for the counselling I think she would have found it impossible – she just couldn't get past my barriers. It was probably the following year before the subject opened up for us and we were able to talk about it, and it's been fine ever since. **99**

HELPFUL TIPS! HELPFUL TIPS! HELPFUL TIPS! HELPFUL

Hints for supporting a breast cancer patient . . .

Friends, family and loved ones have a hugely important role to play in supporting people with breast cancer, but it is not always easy for them to know how best to offer that prop. Here are a few hints on supporting people without swamping them:

- Resist the urge to control or patronise – caring for someone does not have to mean treating them like an infant. Involve them in all decisions wherever possible and respect their wish for solitude and privacy.
- Be yourself as far as possible without adding to their stress – it's OK to express anger, frustration or impatience as you did before they became ill, but also express your love.
- Listen to how they feel without judgement or criticism – if they feel like crying, accept their tears.
- Don't withhold information from them – it isolates people.

- Be their advocate and personal researcher – accompany them to the doctor's and take notes; research treatment options; find support groups.
- Accept offers of help from friends and family – it can take a burden off the patient, and can cement relationships.
- Join a support group or form your own, to give yourself some time off and a chance to unwind and enjoy yourself.

What to tell children

It is important to include children of all ages in the situation and to tell them the truth, though what they are told should be tailored to their age and emotional maturity. Hiding it from them is not a good idea, as it leaves them wide open to making up their own story, which is often much worse than the reality. And they tend to know and understand more than adults allow.

Very young children probably only need to know why their mother is going into hospital or is not her usual self, while slightly older children might understand the situation in terms of good cells and bad cells. All children need to be reassured that they will not be abandoned and that they will be cared for. They need to know, too, that the change in their mother's behaviour is due to her illness and not because she no longer loves them.

Teenagers often find it hard to talk to their parents anyway, and it can be particularly hard for them to be drawn back into the family at a time when they are testing their independence. But that makes it especially important to take time to tell them about what is happening and include them in family decision-making, while avoiding leaning on them too heavily.

The aim should be to let children express their feelings and ask questions about the cancer. How they react will depend on their own personalities and level of emotional maturity, but also on how far their family is supported by relatives and friends and how far their domestic routine of mealtimes and bedtimes has been preserved.

It is a good idea to tell teachers about the situation, so they can lend support at school and keep an eye on how the child is coping.

Apart from shock, grief and feelings of insecurity, the child is likely to be subject to a mixture of powerful emotions, such as anger about being abandoned by the sick parent, irrational guilt that they are somehow responsible for the illness, or fear that the other parent will also develop cancer.

Warning signs that the child needs professional help include: sleep disturbances and nightmares; poor appetite; abnormal fears and 'clingy' behaviour; regression (such as bedwetting); physical and psychological withdrawal; aggressive or destructive behaviour; school refusal.

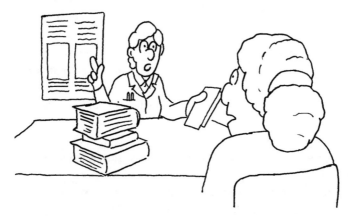

Healthcare staff can help by listening and offering information without overloading.

How can healthcare staff help?

Healthcare staff can also make an enormous difference to the way that emotionally vulnerable breast cancer patients deal with their situation. They can help their patients to minimise their distress and anxiety by dealing sensitively with them, and should:

- Use plain language in a sympathetic way – avoiding both vague euphemisms and brutally frank statements.
- Listen to what the patient says.
- Be alert to verbal and non-verbal cues, such as body language and facial expression.
- Offer information about the cancer and its treatment, without overloading.
- Allow the patient to contribute to decisions about treatment if she or he wishes to.
- Allow the patient to show their emotional distress.
- Give some realistic hope, but no false reassurances.
- Refrain from giving predictions about the cancer's future progress.
- Try to provide continuity of care, where possible, with a few key doctors and nurses.

Most people say their experience of healthcare staff is very positive, but it isn't always the big things that make an impact on patients who are feeling vulnerable.

Molly was grateful to one young doctor for giving her a realistic account of her prognosis:

> ❝The year after my treatment ended a registrar said, 'You've done quite well and rather better than we thought you might.' I can still picture it. He wasn't a particularly charismatic chap, but I found that very helpful actually because it was realistic – he wouldn't have said it if he hadn't meant it.❞

Jill felt positively protected and enriched by her encounters with hospital staff:

> ❝I was in hospital for 11 days and didn't really want to leave. I had flowers and friends and nurses around me and felt positively loved and cared for . . . The chemotherapy sister was a very lovely friendly person who had to face an endless stream of the scared and depressed, encouraging us all to see the brighter side of things.❞

Polly, a qualified doctor, was surprised to find that she didn't want the responsibility for making important decisions about her own treatment and has come away with some ideas about how healthcare professionals can help:

> ❝Nobody assumed I knew anything, which was nice. The one thing I did feel surprised about – because medicine nowadays is all about patient choice and you have to make decisions for yourself – I didn't want to make any decisions. Having medical knowledge, I can go on the internet and look on my medical databases and find as much information as I wanted but I just felt greatly relieved when anybody told me what to do because I really didn't want the responsibility of making the decision. Health professionals have all been very good, but I think it's just knowing you can contact them when you need to, saying – If you've got some more questions and you want to phone me up you can – that's really helpful.❞

Some healthcare professionals, however, can be quite hostile to people who choose not to take their advice. Perhaps they should step back and let their patients make the decisions.

Trish, who chose to reject some of her health advisers' advice, said:

> ❝My consultant is really understanding and supportive of the fact that I chose not to have chemotherapy and tamoxifen and has never made me feel that I have been taking the wrong decision. But there are problems

in trying to stand up to the team – of having to explain why I don't want it. I have no idea why I don't want it! Although they are very supportive and understanding, they do come over as quite critical ... After I had spoken to my consultant to say I didn't want tamoxifen – as I was leaving the nurse handed me a box of tamoxifen. That was distressing. It would be lovely if they could have totally impartial (advisers) – saying, these are the options you can take, these are the people you can call. **"**

Summary

- Friends and relatives can be a major source of support, but many of the observations about the impact of cancer are as true for them as for the patient.

- It is important to include children of all ages in the situation and to tell them the truth, geared to their level of understanding, and offer them reassurance that they will not be abandoned.

- Healthcare staff can make an enormous difference to patients' well-being and minimise their distress by dealing sensitively with them.

What are the treatment options?

Overview

Many people with breast cancer want to take an active part in deciding what treatment they will have, so it's important to know what the options are, and why one treatment is favoured over another. This chapter looks at the different alternatives for treatment and the reasons why one treatment might be preferred over another. It explains what the doctor means by 'grade' and 'stage' of cancer, why some are described as 'oestrogen positive' and why these are important pointers to the most effective treatment. It also looks at clinical trials and the pros and cons of taking part in them.

Treatment options

There are several treatment options, which will be covered in detail in the next three chapters. These are:

- Surgery (see Chapter 8 for more details and Chapter 9 on breast reconstruction).
- Radiotherapy (see Chapter 10).
- Chemotherapy (see Chapter 11).
- Hormonal therapy (see Chapter 12).
- Immunotherapy [biological therapy] (see Chapter 12).

Treatments

Treatments are *local* or *systemic*. Surgery and radiotherapy (or 'radiation therapy') are *local* treatments that are used to remove, destroy or control the cancer cells in a *specific area*. Chemotherapy, hormonal and biological therapy are *systemic* treatments that are used to destroy or control cancer cells *throughout the body* – the 'system'.

The surgeon will discuss a possible treatment plan with the patient once the diagnosis has been made. Sometimes the surgeon will advise just one form of treatment, and sometimes a combination of treatments. But it isn't always possible to make a definite diagnosis and therefore a definite plan before the operation, because the lump and some of the lymph nodes need to be removed and examined under a microscope to determine how aggressive the cancer is and how far it has spread. Depending on the results of tests on both lump and lymph nodes, after the operation, there might need to be further surgery.

The primary treatment for breast cancer is usually surgery, often combined with radiation. *Adjuvant therapy* is treatment that is given to supplement the primary treatment in order to increase the chances of a cure and could include chemotherapy, radiotherapy and/or hormonal therapy.

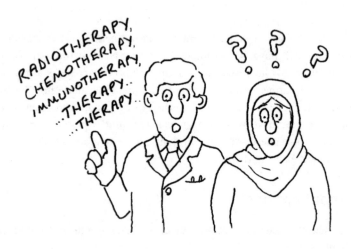

How does the doctor decide what treatment I should have?

In order to make the treatment as effective as possible doctors want to know:

- The stage of the tumour.
- The size of the tumour and where it is in the breast.
- If it has spread within the breast.
- If there is cancer in the lymph nodes in the armpit.

- If the cancer has spread to other parts of the body (metastisised).
- The patient's age and whether she is pre- or post-menopausal.
- Whether the cancer cells depend on female hormones (oestrogen and progesterone) for growth. If so, they are described as oestrogen-positive or progesterone-positive and can be treated by hormonal therapy such as the drug tamoxifen.
- The patient's personal preference.

The treatment options, therefore, depend on a number of things. But the most important factors are the grade and stage of the disease.

What does the doctor mean by 'grade' and 'stage' of cancer?

The doctor will describe a tumour in two ways once it has been removed, examined and classified by a pathologist. One way is by grade – which describes the appearance of tumour cells under the microscope and indicates how fast the tumour is likely to grow and its tendency to spread; and the other is by stage – which is a way of describing how far it has progressed.

The pathologist who examines the tumour will assign it to Grade 1, 2 or 3, according to the kinds of cells that have been identified in it. Grade 1 tumours consist of relatively slow-growing cancer cells that look very much like normal cells and are called 'well-differentiated' cells. Grade 2 are 'moderately differentiated' and more aggressive than Grade 1 cancers. Grade 3 cells are more abnormal in appearance, described as 'poorly differentiated', and are the fastest growing.

The 'stage' – ranging from 0 to IV – is based on the size and type of the tumour, whether it is early or advanced, how aggressive the cancer is and whether it has spread to the lymph nodes or to other organs in the body.

Although the stage and grade of a cancer are different, a combination of the two categories helps the doctor to decide on the most appropriate form of treatment. For instance, if a fast-growing, aggressive Grade 3 cancer is caught at a very early stage, it can have a better outlook than a slow-growing Grade 1 cancer that is not found until after it has spread.

The stages are:

Stage 0 (early stage)

- No actual tumour has been found – as in DCIS or LCIS (see Chapter 2) – and there are no signs of spread to lymph nodes or tissue beyond the breast.

Stage I (early stage)

- The tumour is no more than 2 cm.
- It has not spread to the lymph nodes in the armpit.
- The cancer has not spread to other parts of the body.

Stage II (early stage)

- The tumour is no more than 2 cm but has spread to the lymph nodes in the armpit.
- The tumour is between 2 cm and 5 cm and might or might not have spread to the lymph nodes in the armpit.
- The tumour is larger than 5 cm, but has not spread to the lymph nodes in the armpit.
- The cancer has not spread anywhere else.

Stage III (advanced stage)

- The tumour is more than 5 cm.
- The lymph nodes in the armpit are affected.
- The cancer has not spread elsewhere.

Stage IV (advanced stage)

- The tumour can be any size.
- The cancer has spread to other parts of the body, most commonly the bones, lungs, liver or brain. Or it has spread locally to the skin and lymph nodes above the collarbone.

What are hormone receptor tests?

If the biopsy reveals cancer, it is important that the tumour is also given hormone receptor tests to show whether the cancer cells depend on hormones to grow. Some cancers grow faster in the presence of the female hormone oestrogen, and are called oestrogen receptor positive (ER+) cancers. Some respond in a similar way to the female hormone progesterone and are known as progesterone receptor positive (PR+) cancers. Some respond to either hormone (ER+/PR+), while others do not respond to hormones at all. About three-quarters of post-menopausal breast cancer cases are oestrogen-sensitive.

Those patients whose cancers depend on hormones to grow are more likely to respond to hormonal treatments such as tamoxifen and anastrozole (see Chapter 12), which are notably successful in preventing the return of breast cancers. Having a tumour that is not dependent on hormones to grow does not mean that the chances of cure are worse, just that the treatment will be different.

Is surgery always the first thing that follows diagnosis?

Surgery usually comes first in the list of treatment options, but not always: sometimes tumours are treated with chemotherapy or hormonal therapy to shrink them before surgery, and to suppress the cancerous cells' ability to multiply.

Many women with Stage I breast cancer have the option of breast-sparing surgery followed by radiotherapy and/or hormonal therapy. Sometimes – if the tumour is behind the nipple or the breast is very small – they are advised to have a mastectomy. Sometimes women with Stage I and most with Stage II breast cancer will also be recommended to have chemotherapy to treat the whole body and to prevent metastases and to stop the cancer returning.

Women with Stage III breast cancer usually have both local treatment (surgery and/or radiotherapy) to remove or destroy the cancer in the breast, and systemic treatment (chemotherapy, hormonal therapy or both) to stop it spreading throughout the body.

Those with Stage IV breast cancer are usually given chemotherapy and/or hormonal therapy to shrink the tumour or destroy cancer cells throughout the body. They might also have surgery or radiotherapy to control the cancer in the breast or in other parts of the body.

It is important to remember, though: no operation or procedure can be done without the patient's consent, so if there are any objections to the treatment being offered, it is important to tell the doctor and ask if another treatment is available. And patients do not need to make a decision right away. They should take time to think about their options – to go away and find out more about the treatments, discuss the issues with family and friends, or just sit and think about what they really want. Some women feel they want to keep their breast at all costs; others feel that once it has had cancer in it they would feel happier to have it removed completely. If the cancer is too big or in the centre of the breast, it might only be possible to treat by removing the whole breast.

Some people feel that if the cancer is too far advanced to give them a good chance of being cured, they would rather not subject their body and emotions to the stresses and strains of chemotherapy or radical surgery.

Gwen, who was 59 when she was diagnosed, did not have to face the choice, but says she feels that, having seen others close to her suffer from the effects of chemotherapy she thinks she would choose to take a chance:

❝I'm not sure how I'd respond if it came to it, because I desperately want to live, but at the moment – in remission – I feel that if I found the cancer had spread and there really wasn't much chance of a cure I'd opt for some sort of diet change or something less drastic than chemo. I saw what it did to a close friend, who died from liver cancer, and it seemed to make his last few months a misery – all to no purpose. With hindsight, it might have been better to accept it.**❞**

Box 3.	Some questions to ask your doctor before starting treatment.

- What are my treatment choices?
- What are the benefits of each kind of treatment?
- What are the possible risks and side effects of each treatment?
- Are there any new clinical trials that would be appropriate for me?

Listen to your doctor's reasons for recommending your course of treatment. Once you know what they are, you might feel happier about the decision. If you are still not convinced, you can ask for your test results and X-rays to be supplied to another specialist for a second opinion. It will take time to arrange, so your treatment will be delayed for a while, but most doctors are happy to do this for you.

Jill, who was 44 when she was diagnosed eight years ago, was not happy with her surgeon's recommendations and wanted a second opinion. She says:

❝I was so upset about the idea of losing my breast that I asked if there was any other operation I could have. I saw another surgeon who said, 'We can shrink the tumour with chemo then remove the lump, but you are delaying things by going on this aggressive kind of chemo. But it can be done.' I went home and my nine-year-old son said, 'What are you mucking about at? Everyone knows if you have cancer you have it cut out.' I went in on the Monday and had it done. They took my lymph glands out and found cancer in all of them. It was on its move already. I feel very, very lucky it hadn't got into my bloodstream.**❞**

The doctor or patient might also ask about taking part in a clinical trial, in which new treatments or new treatment techniques are tested out.

Clinical trials

Clinical trials are studies conducted by medical researchers to find out if a new treatment or technique is safe, if it has any side effects and if it is more effective than the current standard treatment. Those for breast cancer look at things like different types of surgery, varying doses of radiotherapy, new drugs, new chemotherapy doses and treatment schedules, and better ways of reducing the side effects of treatments. There are also clinical trials concerned with preventing cancer.

Every new treatment has to go through three phases before it is accepted as the new standard way to manage a condition. Phase 1 trials are the first step in testing out new drugs or treatments on people, after laboratory research that suggests they are promising. These trials are usually small and often recruit people with advanced cancer who have had all the available treatment, but who might benefit from a new regime. They are used to test out the safety of the new treatment, the appropriate dose for new drugs and the possible side effects.

Almost three-quarters of phase 1 trials go on to be tested in phase 2 trials, where the treatment is studied with a slightly larger group of people to find out more about its efficacy, side effects and dosage.

If a phase 2 trial shows the treatment could be as good as or better than standard treatment, it moves to phase 3.

Phase 3 trials usually involve many more people in order to test and compare the treatments as thoroughly and widely as possible, and to expose even quite small differences between them. Phase 3 trials are usually randomised, which means that the people who take part are put into groups at random, generally by a computer. There are at least two groups, sometimes three. Each group is given a different treatment – one of which will be the standard treatment that is given to people who are not in the trial. Those having standard treatment are called the 'control group' and a randomised trial that has a control group is called a 'randomised control trial'. If there is a third group it is sometimes used to test a variation of the new treatment and sometimes is given a placebo (a dummy treatment which looks exactly like the new treatment but has no physical effect, e.g. a tablet of flour and water). But cancer clinical trials usually compare a new treatment with the standard treatment given to people not in the trial and rarely use placebos. All clinical trials have to be agreed by scientists who are independent of the study and then approved by the hospital's research ethics committee. One of the ethics committee's duties is to make sure that the likely benefits of the new treatment are greater than the probable drawbacks, and a trial involving a placebo for a cancer patient would probably not be given the committee's approval. The committee also has the responsibility for ensuring that the trial is well planned, the information for patients is clear and comprehensive and the researchers have arranged insurance cover for compensation if anything should go wrong.

The discoveries from research conducted in this way have led to significant changes in the way that breast cancer is treated. For instance, randomised trials demonstrated some years ago that women with a relatively small cancer were just as likely to be cured if they had a breast-saving lumpectomy followed by radiotherapy, as if they had the whole breast removed.

By law, patients who take part in clinical trials must be fully consulted beforehand. They must be given a full explanation of the purpose of the study, why they are considered suitable, and its implications for their treatment. On the plus side: they might be the first to benefit from improved treatment methods not available anywhere else; their care will be more closely monitored (for instance with blood tests or CT scans); and they will be making a contribution to the advancement of medical knowledge. On the minus side there are risks attached to unknown techniques, of which they should be aware before agreeing to participate. And while some people find the extra check-ups provide reassurance, for others it increases the worry.

Jill was worried that the trial might leave her worse off and decided to turn it down:

> **"**I was offered the opportunity to take part in a clinical trial because I had a second degree cancer, which was on the move and was directly related to my ovaries. I felt pressurised to take part because research has to be carried out for the greater good. But the trial involved taking pills which could be a new drug, the tried and tested tamoxifen or a placebo. After much thought, I decided to go with the best known available drug at that time, which was tamoxifen.
>
> They also asked me to consider an aggressive chemotherapy similar to that given to leukaemia patients. Your bone marrow is removed, they zap you with the chemicals, then inject bone marrow cells back into you so that the bone marrow grows again, free of cancer. Problems arise if the bone marrow cells don't take or if you get an infection whilst your resistance is very low. You stay in intensive care for weeks whilst this is happening and then afterwards you have to be careful about travelling on the tube or going to busy, smoky places with loads of germ-ridden people.
>
> I remember getting tearful and upset and asking [the surgeon] sharply, 'Would you give this treatment to your wife?' He considered the answer and finally said, 'Yes, I think I would.' Later, someone told me that his wife had died from breast cancer and that was a major factor in his decision to specialise in this area. I felt a bloody selfish fool. Other people suffer this too – you forget that you're not the only one when your life is threatened by cancer. However, I felt that if my son was to go off to school and bring back a germ, it could kill me. So, it was selfish, but I felt that I had to give myself and my young son the best chance of my survival and I chose to have the accepted best form of treatment.**"**

In 1796 Edward Jenner injected himself with cow pox and later with smallpox on the basis of anecdotal evidence that the cow pox would protect him from developing smallpox. His theory has still not been tested by randomised trials, but the lives of millions of people have been saved. On the other hand, a lot of remedies based on anecdotal evidence make no difference whatever; using treatment based on old wives' tales is risky, and properly controlled research is the only sure way to improve treatment. Patients who decide they want to withdraw from a clinical trial are free to do so at any stage, without giving a reason, and without affecting their right of access to the standard cancer treatment (see Box 4 for suggested questions to ask your doctor).

Box 4. Some questions on clinical trials to ask your doctor.

- Are there any trials that are suitable for my type and stage of cancer?
- What is being tested in this trial and what will the treatment be?
- What treatment will I get if I don't go into the trial?
- Will I have to go for extra tests?
- What side effects are likely?
- Are there any things I won't be allowed to do if I choose to take part?
- What happens if I want to leave?

Summary

- Treatments are either: *local* (such as surgery and radiotherapy) and used to remove, destroy or control the cancer cells in a specific area; or *systemic* (such as chemotherapy, hormonal and biological therapies) that are used to destroy or control cancer cells throughout the body.

- The most important factors in deciding which is the most effective treatment are the grade and stage of the tumour.

- The grade of a tumour describes the type of cancer cells from which it is made, with Grade 1 the slowest-growing and Grade 3 the most abnormal and fastest-growing.

- The stage of cancer is a combination of the size of tumour, whether there is cancer in the lymph nodes and whether the cancer has spread to the rest of the body.

- Breast cancers are described as oestrogen-positive when they grow faster in the presence of the female hormone oestrogen and this means they can be treated with anti-oestrogen drugs like tamoxifen and anastrozole.

- Clinical trials which are used to test out new treatments are divided into phase 1 (the earliest stage to test safe doses and side effects); phase 2 (to find out more about side effects and effective dosage); and phase 3 (where new treatments are compared with the best currently available, usually in randomised controlled trials).

- Patients who take part are closely monitored, might be the first to benefit from new treatment and are helping to further medical knowledge; but there are risks in agreeing to unknown techniques.

Surgery

Overview

Surgery is the most common treatment for breast cancer, but the surgeon will base the decision about which type to recommend on the size of the cancer, where it is in the breast and whether it has spread to any other part of the body. This chapter will describe the different types of surgery and their possible side effects. It will also look at why and when lymph nodes need to be removed and the possible side effects of this, with an explanation of lymphoedema and hints on how to avoid it.

What are the options for surgery?

Surgeons' advice will range from breast-conserving surgery such as a lumpectomy (where just the cancerous lump is removed) or quadrantectomy (a quarter of the breast is removed), to mastectomy (the whole breast is removed) (see Figure 3).

It is important for patients to talk to the doctor before surgery so they understand the reasons why one operation is recommended rather than another (see Box 5 for some of the questions to ask before surgery).

Box 5.	Some questions to ask your doctor before having surgery.

- Which operation do you recommend for me and why?
- Is a lumpectomy an option for me?
- What are the risks of surgery?
- Will my lymph nodes be removed? If so, why and how many?

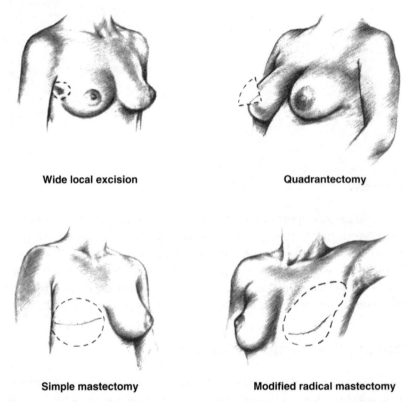

Wide local excision   **Quadrantectomy**

Simple mastectomy   **Modified radical mastectomy**

Figure 3. Different types of surgery. Copyright © 2004 Alexa Rutherford.

- What will my body look like after the operation?
- What will the side effects be?
- If I have a mastectomy will I be able to have plastic surgery to rebuild my breast. If so, how and when can that be done?
- When will I be able to resume my normal activities?

Breast-conserving surgery

The aim of breast-conserving surgery is to minimise the psychological effects to the woman and to give the best cosmetic result, while removing the cancerous cells. Although their breast might not look exactly as it did before surgery, many women prefer to preserve their breast – or as much of it as possible – as long as it is safe to do so. The operations which conserve the breast are:

- Lumpectomy, or wide local excision, where the tumour is removed together with some normal tissue around it (called 'a clear margin'). Some of the lymph nodes under the arm are also removed
- Quadrantectomy – removal of one quarter of the breast and some of the lymph nodes under the arm

But there are other names for the different breast-conserving operations, such as 'partial mastectomy' and 'segmental mastectomy', and surgeons mean different things by the terms. Sometimes, to complicate things further, they use 'lumpectomy' and 'quadrantectomy' to refer to the same thing, and 'wide excision' means a wider clear margin to some surgeons than others. Patients should make sure the surgeon explains precisely how much of the breast he intends to remove and tells them what they will look like after the operation.

The hospital stay is usually around a week for mastectomy, and 5 days, though sometimes less, for lumpectomy.

Lumpectomy

Lumpectomy, followed by radiotherapy, is usually recommended for treating early breast cancer – a small tumour that hasn't spread to the lymph nodes. It might still be recommended where there are multiple tumours, tumours that have migrated to the lymph nodes, or tumours that have spread to other organs in the body, but a systemic treatment such as chemotherapy or hormone therapy will also be prescribed.

Lumpectomy involves the removal of the tumour and a small section of normal breast tissue around it, leaving the breast virtually intact.

Quadrantectomy

A quadrantectomy is similar to a lumpectomy, but up to a quarter of the breast is removed, which means the effects are more noticeable, particularly for women with small breasts.

What are the possible side effects of breast-conserving surgery?

The side effects are usually less drastic after breast-conserving surgery than after a mastectomy and women with small lumps in medium or large breasts look very much the same after the operation as before, except for the scar. But there may be:

- Some loss of sensation in the breast, depending on the size of the lump removed, though there won't be a total loss of feeling as there often is with a mastectomy.
- The breast might be a different size and shape and the nipple position might be changed.
- It might have a dent, or look shrunken or pulled to one side.
- Some women have some sort of pain in the breast area for weeks after surgery, but for others the pain lasts for years.

Mastectomy

Radical mastectomy used to be the standard and only operation for breast cancer until research showed that lumpectomy followed by radiotherapy is just as effective in eradicating the cancer for most women with early stage tumours. In the past, in addition to removing all the breast tissue, mastectomy involved removing the chest muscles and all the lymph nodes up to the collarbone. Today, chemotherapy is usually used to shrink very large tumours before surgery, so this operation is rarely performed. Mastectomy now is much less drastic and refers to a range of operations where as much of the breast tissue as possible is removed, including the nipple, but rarely any of the muscle. The two commonest mastectomy operations are:

- Simple (total) mastectomy, where the whole breast is removed from the collar bone to the edge of the ribs and from the breastbone to the muscle at the back of the armpit, including the nipple and excess skin, but the muscles are not removed. Some of the lymph nodes under the arm might also be removed.
- Modified radical mastectomy (now only used when the cancer is advanced and has spread to the chest muscles) where the whole breast is removed, together with part of the muscle on the chest wall, and some or all the lymph nodes under the arm.

Why is mastectomy sometimes recommended rather than lumpectomy?

Although lumpectomy is suitable for most early stage cancers, mastectomy is often recommended as the most suitable treatment if:

- There is a large lump in a small breast and a lumpectomy would leave a very misshapen breast.
- The tumour is in the middle of the breast, just behind the nipple – where cutting out the lump would mean removing the nipple.
- There is more than one area of cancer in the breast.
- There are areas of DCIS in the rest of the breast.
- The woman is pregnant and radiotherapy would present a danger to her unborn baby.
- The breast has already been treated with radiotherapy.
- The woman has some other health condition (such as collagen vascular diseases like lupus or scleroderma) or chronic lung disease, which makes radiotherapy inadvisable.
- The woman chooses not to have radiotherapy.
- The woman would rather have the whole breast removed.

Many women – though not all – see their breasts as an important part of their sexual identity, and the prospect of losing one or both is something that adds to their distress at the diagnosis of breast cancer (see Chapter 14).

Molly, who was 62 when she was diagnosed in 1989, regarded her breasts as important to the way she viewed herself. She said:

> **❝**One of my nightmares has always been of the possibility of having to have a mastectomy – it filled me with horror ... the first thing I asked when I came round (from the operation) was, 'Have I still got my nipple?' And I had, so I knew I wouldn't have a mastectomy because he wouldn't have bothered saving it if I was going to.**❞**

On the other hand, Kay, who was aged 31 when she was diagnosed with breast cancer in 2001, said she had been less worried about losing her breast than her mother had been 18 months before. Kay said:

> **❝**I think I coped with the mastectomy really well. I find that women who are older are more worried about not having a breast – my mum had it 18 months before I had it, she was 59 and she had to have reconstruction, she couldn't bear to be without a bosom. But with me it didn't affect me in any way. I felt so lucky that I do hairdressing. I've got my hands, I've got my legs, I can do the work, it was a part of the body that wasn't going to be missed. And I probably have had much more fun with my sex life than what I did before. It's not really been a problem ... but I am going to have reconstruction.**❞**

What are the possible side effects of mastectomy?

Mastectomy can have several side effects, some of which last a short time and others which are permanent.

- For a woman with large breasts it can throw her weight out of balance and lead to aches and pains in her neck and back.
- The skin in the area where the breast was removed might be tight.
- The muscles of the arm and shoulder might feel stiff. Some women permanently lose some strength in these muscles, but the loss is temporary for most people, and a physiotherapist can recommend exercises to help.
- There might be some numbness and tingling in the chest, underarm, shoulder and upper arm from nerves damaged during surgery. These feelings often disappear within a few weeks or months, but for some women the numbness is permanent.
- Permanent numbness around the scar, where the breast's nerve supply has been cut. Sometimes the breast area has some sensitivity, but it can be quite uncomfortable, like the tingly sensation when your foot's been asleep and the feeling starts to come back.
- Some women have phantom breast symptoms, such as itchy nipples, which should gradually improve as the brain becomes reprogrammed.

Jill, who had a mastectomy 8 years ago, says her breasts were 'rather enormous' and the loss of one has thrown her weight out of balance:

> **❝**I feel very lop-sided, and at first I would almost stagger to one side when I got out of bed half asleep ... I couldn't lift my arm very freely at first but after a year I was swimming and playing badminton regularly. I don't have as much strength in my right arm as I used to and I find it aches if I am stretching up to hang curtains or decorate. I never use weights on my rare appearances at the gym because I think it would be too much of a strain. However, I can lift my arms up above my head and manage to rock'n'roll when the occasion demands it.**❞**

Lymph gland removal

Examining the lymph nodes will indicate whether the cancer has spread and help the doctor to decide further treatment.

We all have thousands of lymph nodes throughout the body, which act as filters for lymph fluid and help the immune system to fight disease. The lymph nodes under the arm drain lymph fluid from the chest and arm. The surgeon usually removes lymph glands from the armpit (the axilla) during breast cancer surgery, because they are helpful in detecting whether the cancer has spread from its original site. Once the breast surgery has been finished the surgeon begins to remove the lymph nodes. Sometimes all the lymph glands in the armpit are removed (axillary clearance) and sometimes just a few (sampling). The surgeon makes an incision across the armpit and removes a section of fat that usually has 10 to 15 lymph nodes embedded in it, although it can be many more or far fewer. It is hoped, though not certain, that the significant lymph nodes (the ones that are most likely to have cancer) are included in this section. The tissue is sent to a pathologist who examines each node to see if the cancer is present.

Women with DCIS are unlikely to have their nodes removed, because the cancerous cells are entirely enclosed in the breast's ducts.

Sometimes the armpit is also treated with radiotherapy, although this is avoided where possible when the lymph nodes have been removed, as it can increase the risk of lymphoedema (see below for more information).

Sentinel node biopsy

This is still undergoing trial, and is not yet standard treatment. The surgeon injects a small amount of blue dye or radioactive material (or both) into the area around the tumour. As this drains away to the lymph glands the surgeon can identify the first node – the sentinel node – that it reaches. This node, which is the most likely to have cancer if it has spread, can be tracked via the blue lymph vessel (or the gamma counter if a radioactive tracer is used) leading to it. It is then removed – often with the two or three nearest to it as well – and examined. If this node is negative the remaining lymph nodes might not need to be removed.

If the node is positive for cancer the surgeon will either offer a second operation to remove all the lymph nodes under the arm, or radiotherapy to kill any remaining cancerous cells.

Some scientists say that if the technique is found to be effective it will mean that patients whose nodes are clear will no longer need to have all the lymph nodes under the arm removed. But others say that it is not foolproof and provides a false negative in about 5 per cent of cases.

Side effects of lymph gland removal

There are possible complications of the operation to remove lymph glands, some more serious than others:

- Many women find that their armpit is numb after surgery, where the surgeon has cut the nerve that runs through the fat containing the lymph nodes. Most breast surgeons and some general surgeons try to save the nerve, but even when they do it may be stretched and leave the patient with decreased sensation. Sometimes the feeling comes back after a few months, but sometimes there is a permanent patch of numbness. This can make it difficult to shave under the arms safely.

- Sometimes one of the veins in the arm becomes inflamed and very painful, but the condition rarely lasts more than one or two weeks.

- Most women get some swelling under the armpit following surgery, due to the fluid that collects there, but for some it gets to the size of a cricket ball and needs to be drawn off with a needle.

- In the short term, the arm and shoulder on the side of the operation will probably feel sore and stiff and movement is likely to be very restricted in them for some weeks. The physiotherapist or breast care nurse will give the patient exercises to help them regain full movement.

In the longer term, there is a risk of a major complication, a condition called 'lymphoedema' in which the arm swells up and for which, although it can be managed, there is no cure.

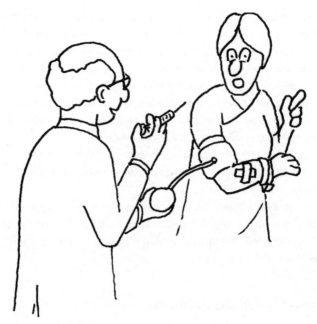

Help of protect your arm from lymphoedema by having injections and tests done on the other arm.

What is lymphoedema and how do I avoid it?

Surgery and radiotherapy to the armpit can interfere with the normal drainage of fluid. The lymph nodes act like a strainer, removing foreign material and bacteria. Scars from surgery in the area can block some of the holes and hinder drainage. This can result in swelling of the arm and hand (called lymphoedema), usually in the arm nearest the affected breast. The swelling can be temporary, but can persist for months, years or even permanently. It can develop immediately after surgery or months, even years, later. Symptoms include a 'tight' feeling in the limb or skin, decreased flexibility in joints, particularly hands and wrists, and persistent swelling. It can be a sign that the cancer has returned.

Acute lymphoedema lasts less than 6 months and is often resolved within a week by keeping the affected limb raised (perhaps with the arm on a pillow when lying down, or in a sling when up and about).

Chronic lymphoedema (that lasts for longer than 6 months) is a serious condition that is very difficult to treat. There is no cure, but specially trained physiotherapists can help in its management.

Complex Decongestive Therapy is an intensive course of treatment that usually lasts from ten days to six weeks and is often beneficial. It includes skin and nail care, daily manual lymphatic drainage, daily multilayer compression bandaging and daily exercises to encourage efficient lymph flow. Unfortunately, very few clinics offer the full CDT and not all the elements are available on the NHS. Contact the Lymphoedema Support Network for details (www.lymphoedema.org, or see 'Useful addresses and contacts' at the back of the book).

Joan was 64 when she had a mastectomy and 13 lymph nodes removed, and was shocked when she developed lymphoedema a year after surgery. She says:

❝My husband had bought me a bangle and it wouldn't go on ... I put it on the other hand and it fitted ... I have no idea what triggered it. They gave me a lot of antibiotics that first year, but it didn't go down. It's swollen all the time and sometimes it's painful, but most of the time I just forget about it. It's about twice the size of the other arm and I have to buy bigger-sized blouses because of the sleeves.

I did have a [pressure] sleeve and a glove, but because I'm right-handed I found it very restrictive ... you're not supposed to wear the sleeve without the glove – it would just push all the swelling into your hand ... I wear them when I'm not expecting to do anything – but you can't cook, obviously, with them on, they're not very hygienic. I can't hang washing up because holding my arm up is too heavy and vacuuming I find a bit difficult, but it doesn't really restrict me doing other things.❞

John started with lymphoedema after developing an infection:

> **"**I had a slight infection in the wound, and having had all my tubes taken out I then had to have them put back in and as a result I now have lymphoedema. I was out in the garden and cutting roses and at the end of the day I found my arm was extremely tired and I was booked into the lymphoedema clinic. I now have the elastic arms and hands, which seem to hold it in trim. Also the lymphoedema sister said if I put some of this special adhesive bandage under my right armpit it helps to support the muscle there. I don't get any pain with it, it's a slight discomfort and I'm conscious of it. If I wear this bit of bandage it's a bit of a pain when you have a shower because you have to dry it with a hairdryer. I must admit I'm not showering quite as often as I used to, but I change that every couple of days and it does seem to help.**"**

No one can accurately predict who will and who won't get lymphoedema, but there are things that can be done to avoid the circumstances that are known to trigger it (see the box for hints on protection from lymphoedema).

HELPFUL TIPS! HELPFUL TIPS! HELPFUL TIPS! HELPFUL

How to help protect your arm from lymphoedema

- Have injections (including chemotherapy), blood tests and blood pressure tests done on the other arm.
- Carry heavy shopping or handbags on the other arm or shoulder.
- Avoid sunburn and burns on your affected arm and hand.
- Avoid cuts when shaving underarms – use an electric shaver.
- Wash cuts promptly, apply antibacterial medication and cover with a plaster or bandage. See your doctor if think you have an infection.
- Wear gloves to protect your hands when gardening and washing up.
- Avoid wearing tight jewellery or elastic cuffs on your affected arm.
- Be careful when manicuring your nails and avoid cutting your cuticles.

- Wear compression garments, such as a special sleeve, when flying, to maintain a constant pressure.

Summary

- Surgery is the most common treatment for breast cancer, and the type recommended is based on where it is in the breast and whether it has spread to anywhere else in the body.

- Options are: breast-conserving surgery to preserve as much of the breast as possible given the need to remove cancerous cells, and means lumpectomy (removal of just the lump) or quadrantectomy (removing a quarter of the breast); otherwise, mastectomy (removing the whole breast including the nipple).

- Lumpectomy, followed by radiotherapy, is usually recommended for treating early-stage cancer and a quadrantectomy is similar, but removes up to a quarter of the breast.

- Mastectomy is a better option than lumpectomy if: there is a large lump in a small breast; the tumour is behind the nipple, there is more than one area of cancer; there are areas of DCIS in the breast; radiotherapy presents a health problem; the woman prefers it.

- Lymph glands are removed as an indicator of whether or not the cancer has spread.

- Sentinel node biopsy is a new procedure that might – when it has been properly tested – eliminate the need to remove more than one or two lymph nodes.

- Lymphoedema is a serious possible side effect of surgical removal of the lymph nodes which can be temporary or permanent; it can happen immediately or years after the operation; it can result in an extreme and irreversible swelling of the arm.

Breast reconstruction or prosthesis?

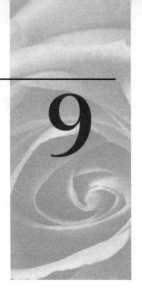

9

Overview

Most women see their breasts as an important part of their femininity and sexual identity, and the loss of one or both adds to the burden of the news that they have cancer. This chapter looks at who is suitable for breast reconstruction, when it can be done and the different types of breast reconstruction that are available. It also considers the use of a prosthesis.

Who chooses to have a breast reconstruction?

Some women feel they want to keep their breast at almost any cost, while others feel that they will only feel safe if it is removed altogether. Some women, who find the prospect of a mastectomy too emotionally painful, might want an immediate breast reconstruction, while others are keen to avoid further surgery and satisfied to wear a prosthesis, or breast form, in the empty side of their bra. Surgeons will discuss the different options for breast reconstruction, and the hospital's breast care nurse or appliance officer will advise on the different types of prosthesis that are available on the NHS and from private suppliers.

Jill is saddened by the loss of her breast, but has rejected the idea of a reconstruction because of the extra surgery:

> **❝**When this happened I just wanted the cancer cut out. They offered to give me a reconstruction but they showed me some pictures and no-one looked like Pamela Anderson. I didn't want to go through any more surgery.**❞**

Who is suitable for breast reconstructive surgery and when can it be done?

Most women could have surgical breast reconstruction after mastectomy, but if it is being considered it is a good idea to discuss the options before surgery so the doctor can assess whether immediate reconstruction is a good idea, or whether it would be better to wait.

If radiation therapy is likely to be necessary, and for patients whose skin healing is impaired – for instance by diabetes or collagen vascular disease – it might be better to wait. If they are fit enough, women can have breast reconstruction at any age, and it can be done years after the mastectomy if they change their original decision.

Breast reconstruction should be done by someone who is experienced in this very specialised type of surgery. Not all breast surgeons carry out reconstruction, but they should be able to advise women on how to find a suitably qualified plastic surgeon in their area. There might be a waiting list for treatment.

What are the options?

The type of reconstruction that the surgeon will recommend depends on factors such as a woman's age and body type, and the type of treatment she has had or might need in the future. Reconstruction will not recreate the lost breast. It will not have natural sensation and usually there will be no nipple. But skilled surgeons can create something that looks like a breast.

The different types of breast reconstruction are:

- An implant under the skin of the breast.
- An implant under the chest muscles.
- Moving skin and muscle from another part of the body.
- Moving skin and fat from another part of the body.

These will now be described.

Breast implants

Under the skin

Breast implants under the skin of the breast are the simplest, most readily available type of breast reconstruction. The surgeon removes the breast tissue, but keeps the skin and nipple. An implant made out of silicone rubber and filled with saline (salt water) or silicone gel is inserted under the skin. This is sometimes favoured by women who have a high risk of cancer and have their breasts removed to prevent it. But some consultants are reluctant to leave the nipple, as the cancer could develop there.

There has been some concern about silicone gel and its possible effect on the body's immune system, and some suggestion that it could cause arthritis or skin conditions. If this is a worry, it might be better to opt for an implant filled with saline. The implant will still be in a silicone rubber casing, but this has not been blamed for any adverse effects. The advantage of saline is that if it leaks it is harmless, but the disadvantage is that it feels more like water than flesh.

Under the chest muscles

Breast implants placed under the chest muscles are only suitable for women with very small breasts, as the skin will not stretch enough to take a large implant. It is also not suitable for women who have had radiotherapy following the mastectomy, or for those who have had a radical mastectomy, in which the chest muscles are removed. This kind of implant tends to stay firm, while the other breast might not and it won't gain or lose weight with the rest of the body. It is a good choice for women who have had bilateral mastectomies and who are happy with small breasts.

Tissue expansion

With tissue expansion, the skin and chest muscles are slowly stretched over a period of 4 to 6 months, to take an implant. An empty inflatable bag is placed behind the muscle and everything is sewn up, then the bag is inflated gradually over the course of 4 to 6 months by injecting saline into the bag through a valve until the breast shape is the right size, when it is replaced with a silicone or saline implant in a second operation. The disadvantage is that the reconstructed breast might be higher and might not look much like the other breast.

Moving skin and muscle from another part of the body

Flap reconstruction

An alternative to implants or tissue expansion is to have flap reconstruction (see Figure 4). With this, the surgeon makes use of the patient's own skin, fat and muscle to form the new breast. This is done either by cutting flaps in which the muscle and overlying tissues are rotated into place without interrupting the original blood supply to the muscle, or by detaching the tissue and sewing the blood vessels in the new location to establish a new blood flow.

The flap can be taken:

- from the abdomen – a TRAM (transverse rectus abdominus muscle) flap
- from the back – latissimus dorsi
- from the buttocks – a gluteal flap

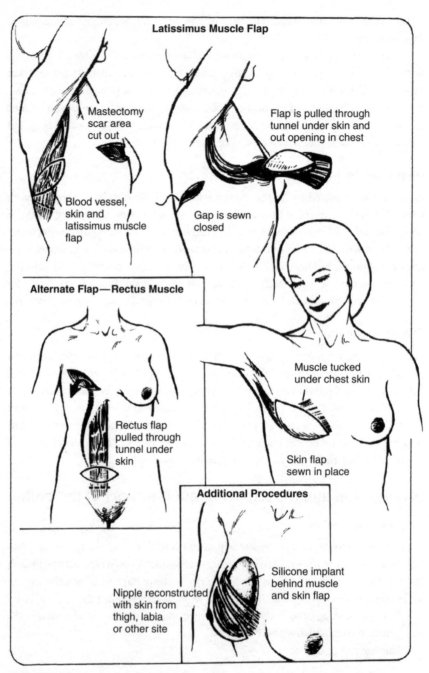

Figure 4. Breast reconstruction techniques. From Brown and Leffall, *100 Questions and Answers about Breast Cancer* (2003) Jones & Bartlett Publishers, Sudbury, MA. www.jbpub.com. Reprinted with permission.

From the abdomen – the TRAM flap is also known as the 'tummy tuck'. One of two muscles from the abdomen, together with skin and fat, is moved to the chest and then shaped like a breast. The patient will have a scar across the lower abdomen, plus a scar on her chest, and the area where the muscle was removed may be weakened, leaving her at greater risk of a hernia in the future.

From the back – the latissimus dorsi is a large, fan-shaped muscle in the back, under the shoulder blade. The surgeon can use this to make a new breast shape from the fat and muscle, but it usually also needs an implant under the new muscle so that the reconstruction matches the other breast. There will be a scar on the back and on the breast.

From the buttocks – the surgeon removes part of the skin and fat from the buttocks and grafts it on to the chest. The success of this operation depends on an adequate blood supply reaching the tissues and has a higher risk of failure than the latissimus dorsi.

DIEP reconstruction – 'Deep Inferior Epigastric Perforator' is the name of the blood vessels involved in this new technique. This is similar to the TRAM flap operation, but the muscle is left in place, while skin and fat is removed, together with its own blood supply to ensure its survival in its new location.

Nipples

Nipples can be reconstructed from the darker skin from the inner thigh and stitched on to the breast – usually a few months after the original surgery to ensure it is in the right place.

If the woman opts for breast reconstruction at the same time as the mastectomy, it could be possible for her to preserve her own nipple by having it stitched to the abdomen or inner thigh then grafted to the new breast shape once it has settled down.

Tattooing a nipple shape is an alternative to surgery.

Prostheses

For women who decide they don't want further surgery but would like to maintain the symmetry of two breasts, a prosthesis – an artificial breast form – is available on the NHS or privately for about £100. After a mastectomy the NHS patient is given a lightweight foam prosthesis which is specially designed to be worn immediately after the operation when the area is particularly sensitive. When the wound is fully healed a permanent prosthesis will be provided. The prostheses come in all shapes, sizes and colours and are constantly improving in texture. Some fit inside the bra, while others are attached to the skin – with glue, Velcro tape or ready sticky-backed. (See 'Useful addresses and contacts' at the back of the book for organisations that can help.)

Jill is still searching for the perfect prosthesis – and a sexy bra. She says:

> **"**I've just got used to wearing a prosthesis like I wear my glasses. It feels very life-like but I have to have a really heavy one (size 10) so I'm not really a suitable candidate for some of the new stick-on ones. I enjoy swimming so I've bought a special one which is not quite so heavy, with a hollowed out back, that dries quickly. The weight always makes my bra dig into me and I'm always looking for a bra which fits that isn't white, black or skin tone. The main department stores are full of beautiful colours but none of them are ever suitable for me. Most boned bras push you up and together to form a cleavage which is just what I can't have. So I need a minimiser type of bra which just gives me a supportive shape – but they are always very mumsy and usually white. Even after surgery I would like to look pretty and sexy – but at least I'm around to be able to complain!**"**

Summary

- Most women would be eligible for surgical breast reconstruction after a mastectomy, but it should be discussed with the surgeon before surgery to determine whether it could be done immediately or whether it would be better to wait.

- Breast reconstruction should be done by a specialist breast surgeon or plastic surgeon, but there might be a waiting list.

- A reconstructed breast will not have natural sensation and there will be no nipple, although one can be constructed or tattooed on at a later date.

- Breasts can be reconstructed by inserting implants, by moving skin and muscle or skin and fat from another part of the body.

- Breast prostheses (artificial breast forms) are available from the NHS and private suppliers in all shapes, sizes and colours and can be attached in a variety of ways.

Radiotherapy

Overview

Radiotherapy (also called radiation therapy) has been found to be an effective way of destroying breast cancer cells lurking after surgery and its widespread use has led to fewer mastectomies and more breast-conserving operations. This chapter looks at what it is and which patients are suitable for treatment. It explains what happens in simulation and why it is used to plan the treatment. It reports what happens and how it feels in a radiotherapy session and describes the commoner short- and long-term side effects. There is also an explanation of the less common brachytherapy (internal radiotherapy).

What is it?

Radiotherapy uses radiation, usually high-energy X-rays, to treat the cancer and stop it growing. The radiation is similar to that used for taking an X-ray picture, but the beams are very much stronger and are aimed at the cancer very precisely. If there are any microscopic cancer cells left in the breast after surgery, this should destroy them.

Radiotherapy alone is not usually seen as a method of curing breast cancer. On its own it is unlikely to destroy large lumps of cancerous cells, but it can often wipe out any lingering clusters of tumour cells left behind when all visible cancer has been removed. It is nearly always recommended after lumpectomy, to reduce the risk of the cancer returning in the same breast.

Radiotherapy is also sometimes given after a mastectomy where there is a high risk of recurrence. It is not usually given to the armpit if all the lymph glands there have been removed as it can increase the risk of developing lymphoedema.

Treatment usually starts two to four weeks after surgery to make sure that everything has healed and it is not too painful to keep the arm raised above the head (though chemotherapy would normally be placed between surgery and radiotherapy if needed). The decision about how much radiation to give and for how long is based on the grade, type and staging of the tumour. It can come from a machine outside the body (external) or less commonly, internally, from implants (internal radiation or brachytherapy).

External radiotherapy

Most radiotherapy departments give treatment daily on 4 or 5 days each week, leaving weekends free, over a period, typically, of 6 weeks, though there are studies currently exploring whether the same treatment can be given in higher doses in just 3 weeks.

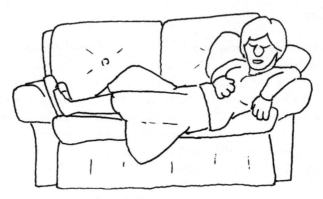

Fatigue is a common side effect of radiotherapy.

What is 'simulation'?

On the first visit to the radiotherapy department, the patient will be taken for simulation, when the treatment will be planned. The simulator replicates the radiotherapy machine, but uses the same energy as a chest X-ray machine and gives normal X-ray doses, but not treatment doses. Radiographers use the pictures from the simulator, together with any scans, to plan precisely how much irradiation should be given from different angles to maximise the effect on the cancer and minimise the damage to other normal tissues and cells and to the underlying lungs or heart. Computerised models can work out the best direction of irradiation beams and doses to be given.

Once the treatment site is lined up, the radiographer will mark the target area with felt tip pens, which will wash off, and one or two tiny pinprick tattoos which are permanent, and which are used as a guide to ensure that the irradiation is delivered in exactly the right direction. The tattoo is also useful as a marker for future reference, to make sure a radiographer knows the patient has had radiation in that area, as you must only have radiotherapy once on any given spot. The simulation takes from half an hour to two hours and is painless. Nevertheless, by this stage, some people start to feel weary of the whole process.

Molly's experience illustrates this. Aged 62 when she was first diagnosed, Molly had had a lumpectomy but no radiotherapy. A year later another lump appeared in the same breast and she went for radiotherapy. She said:

> **“**I began to think my body wasn't my own. One morning when I went to the hospital I was examined by three different doctors and had a mammogram. And after they'd marked me up – gentian violet lines all over – a friend rang me and I was trying to tell her what I felt like and she said, it sounds a bit like a carcass in a butcher's shop, which is exactly right. Radiographers are all very pleasant, but it's a conveyor belt.**”**

How does radiotherapy feel, and what happens in a treatment session?

Radiotherapy does not cause any pain or any sensation at all. There is no heat, light or sound (other than a whooshing sound when the machine is switched on).

For the treatment, the patient removes her upper clothing (see the box for hints on precautions to take during radiotherapy treatment). The radiographer positions her on the treatment table holding on to an armrest, where she must stay completely still for a few minutes (1 to 5 minutes at most), though breathing normally. The radiographer then goes into a nearby room with a glass window to operate the radiation machines, which will move around during treatment. The radiation is given from a number of different angles, so the therapist will come back in, re-position the patient and leave again. The two can continue to talk to each other via a microphone installed in the room and the treatment can be halted if necessary.

Some people like to hear music during the few minutes it takes, and many hospitals arrange for it to be piped into the treatment room.

Gwen, who started radiotherapy 5 weeks after a lumpectomy, found the music pleasantly distracting. She said:

> **“**The radiotherapy machine made a whooshing noise when it was switched on, then they played Louis Armstrong's 'What a Wonderful World' and I stared at a poster of some peaceful meadow scene pasted on the ceiling – all the while counting 'one and, two and . . .' for about two minutes. I can't remember exactly how long now, but the end of the session usually coincided with my counting. Good job I like Louis Armstrong!**”**

Most people are relieved after the first treatment because they see how painless and easy the actual treatments are.

Some people continue to work in between treatments, while others ask for shorter working hours or time off during this period.

Gwen, who reports having few side effects from radiotherapy, took time off, but says she could probably have continued to work:

> **"**I had six weeks' treatment and took the whole time off work, though some people go in, I believe. In fact, for most of that time I felt a complete fraud because I felt so well. I live in south London and was treated at St Thomas's, which meant that I walked along the Embankment, past the London Eye every morning in the sunshine, and I often used to have tears in my eyes because it was so beautiful and I was so glad to be alive. Plus, the staff were so kind and understanding when I got there.**"**

Kay had a mastectomy followed by chemotherapy then radiotherapy after that, and also found the radiotherapy trouble-free. She said:

> **"**Radiotherapy – that was very easy. I did a clinical trial for them and actually managed to get a 3-week course, very intense, it normally goes on for five weeks. It takes more time taking your clothes off than having the treatment itself. It's not painful and my skin didn't burn up.**"**

HELPFUL TIPS! HELPFUL TIPS! HELPFUL TIPS! HELPFUL

Precautions to take during radiotherapy

For the skin:

- Use unscented soaps.
- Bathe in lukewarm water.
- Don't use any: deodorants; talcum powder; skin cream (though E45 or aqueous creams are routinely advised in between sessions); sun block or other substances on the skin, they can all interact with the radiation and it's important to avoid them.
- Wear loose, soft cotton clothing over the treated area.
- Don't scratch, rub or scrub treated skin.
- Cover the skin to protect it from the sun.

Boost

After the radiotherapy course has been completed there is usually a 'boost' – an extra dose of radiation aimed at the area where the tumour was or the scar where it was removed. The boost is usually given by a machine that emits an electron beam which does not penetrate very deeply.

What are the common side effects and how can I deal with them?

Most patients have no major side effects while they are having treatment, though they often have some minor – usually short-lived – problems. And some have none. It does not mean their treatment is not working just as effectively if there are no side effects – it just means they are fortunate.

Jill had no major side effects, and rather enjoyed the experience. She said:

> ❝The radiotherapy didn't seem to hurt me. My skin went slightly pink, but I rather felt I was being looked after, the radiographers were lovely, and it was quite nice to chat to the other women there who were going through the same thing.❞

Short-term side effects

Short-term effects include skin irritation, redness and itching, which are like mild sunburn, and are more common in fair-skinned people. When skin reactions occur, they usually start in the second or third week of treatment and disappear within 4 to 6 weeks.

Some patients lose their appetite and have difficulty with their digestive system during treatment. It is important to make sure they are getting proper nutrition and it might be useful to take a vitamin and mineral supplement during this time.

Fatigue – ranging from mild to severe – is a fairly common complaint. It can last for 4 to 6 weeks after treatment ends or occasionally for several months. It can even start after the treatment has finished.

If fatigue is a problem it is probably a good idea to cut back on stressful activities if at all possible and a good idea to:

- Make sure to eat a balanced diet and consider taking a vitamin and mineral supplement, at least for a few months.
- Take some mild exercise, such as a short walk – matching activity to energy levels.

Kay, who was 32 when she was having her treatment, was quite tired, but not so exhausted as after the rigours of chemotherapy:

> 66The only thing, it was extremely tiring going backwards and forwards to the hospital every day. You felt exhausted but not in an uncomfortable way of feeling ill like the chemotherapy, just really tiring, you feel as though your body's been through a lot. But it goes very quickly, that's the only thing I can say. 99

Molly, aged 63 when she had her radiotherapy, was already feeling drained when her treatment started and found that it was quite an ordeal. She said:

> 66I'd had both hips replaced a few years before and the right one was getting a bit rocky so I was on crutches when I had to go for radiotherapy. The weather was lovely – it was April – so I measured my progress by how far I could walk – feeling very depleted, very weary, tiring very quickly. 99

All the emotions that invariably accompany a diagnosis of breast cancer, such as fear, anger and sadness can sometimes lead to depression. If it happens, though, it is usually after treatment is over – possibly because the treatment gives a feeling of doing something to fight the cancer but once it ends there is a sense of letdown.

Long-term side effects

In the long term, some women find that the skin of the treated breast is reddened and either thickened or thinned for a year or more after treatment ends, and sometimes the changes can be permanent. The nipple may lose some of its pigmentation and internal scarring may make the breast feel firmer. It can result in the breast either becoming slightly bigger or slightly smaller. There may be sharp, shooting pains from time to time.

Gwen's skin started to react quite soon after treatment started, but over the course of the next two years it gradually returned to something like normal. She said:

> 66My breast went quite pink quite early on. I was warned that it would probably be a bit discoloured for ever, but it looks more or less normal now after two years – though the nipple's paler. And it's firmer – which must be good news! 99

Women who have had lumpectomies followed by radiotherapy sometimes develop mastitis as their skin is more delicate and prone to cuts and some of the lymph nodes, which help to fight infection, have been removed. The breast infection is usually accompanied by a fever and headache and should respond to antibiotics. But an infection will either get better or worse: if the condition does neither, the symptoms could be masking cancer and must be investigated further.

More seriously, but extremely rarely, radiation can cause second cancers. These don't occur until at least 5 years after radiotherapy and are very uncommon. During radiation of the breast a bit of the heart and lung can be affected and some studies show that people who had radiation therapy for cancer in their left breasts some years ago had an increased rate of heart disease. Studies of the improved radiotherapy machines which give much more precise treatment, appear to show that there is virtually no increased risk of heart problems following radiotherapy now. Some people develop a persistent cough, however, following treatment.

Internal radiotherapy (brachytherapy)

Internal radiotherapy (brachytherapy) is not commonly used for breast cancer, but when it is used it is usually for treating deep-seated or very large cancers, where external irradiation might not reach the whole cancer. It can be delivered by inserting radioactive material directly into the breast, via a small sealed metal tube or metal wires. Temporary implants are the most common method of internal radiotherapy used to treat breast cancer.

The advantage is that the irradiation is targeted precisely and in greater concentration than is possible with external radiotherapy. The disadvantage is that some cancer cells might escape unless the radioactive materials are implanted extremely accurately, so brachytherapy is usually given in conjunction with external radiotherapy.

With this type of radiotherapy the woman will stay in hospital with the implants in place for several days. She will be isolated from other people while the radiation is working and visitors' contact will be limited. The implants will be removed with a local anaesthetic before she goes home.

Research suggests that this treatment, combined with external radiotherapy, could be more effective for locally advanced cancers than radical surgery.

Summary

- Radiation, which is also called radiation therapy, uses high-energy X-rays to wipe out any lingering tumour cells left behind in the breast tissue after surgery but is not helpful in destroying large lumps of cancer.

- Radiotherapy is nearly always recommended after lumpectomy, but sometimes also following a mastectomy.

- Radiotherapy can come from a machine outside the body or from implants in the body (brachytherapy).

- Treatment is usually given every day for 5 days, leaving weekends free, over a period of 3 to 6 weeks.

- Simulation is the first stage of radiotherapy, when radiographers use a replica radiotherapy machine which uses only low-energy radiation to plan precisely the angles and amount of irradiation to the breast. Once calculated, the target area is given a pinprick tattoo.

- Radiotherapy sessions are completely painless and last for only a few minutes each.

- Short-term side effects include skin irritation, redness and itching.

- Long term – very rarely – it can cause a second cancer, and some studies have shown that women receiving radiotherapy on their left breast have a higher rate of heart disease.

Chemotherapy

Overview

'Chemotherapy,' according to the dictionary, means the use of chemicals to treat disease. But we usually use the word only to refer to the cytotoxic chemicals that kill cells and are used to treat cancer. This chapter looks at why chemotherapy is used for some people with breast cancer but not for others, and at how it works. It also outlines the common side effects and gives hints on how to cope with them.

What is chemotherapy?

Chemotherapy uses anti-cancer drugs to kill or damage cancer cells, either in the original tumour or where they have spread through the bloodstream into the rest of the body.

One reason why cancerous cells are dangerous is that they reproduce at high speed. Generally, the drugs used in chemotherapy are cytotoxic (which means 'poisonous to cells'). They kill rapidly dividing cancer cells and therefore the cancer. But they also poison rapidly dividing normal cells – hair, digestive tract, and bone marrow cells, for instance – which is why they often cause side effects such as hair loss, loss of appetite, sore mouth, diarrhoea and fatigue. The bone marrow produces red blood cells (which have haemoglobin that carries oxygen around the body), white blood cells (that fight infections), and platelets (that help to clot the blood to prevent bleeding); so the effects of injuring it are bound to be potentially serious.

Chemotherapy slows the production of bone marrow down, but it is obviously important not to stop it altogether so this is one reason why chemotherapy is usually given in cycles, with treatment sessions followed by a few weeks of recovery time, to allow the body time to repair itself. The interval between treatments also helps to ensure that all the cancerous cells are killed, not just those that were at the right stage when the drug was first given. And it gives the patient a welcome break, to ward off depression or emotional exhaustion.

Blood counts are taken before treatment and at regular intervals once it is under way as an indicator of the bone marrow's recovery rate, which helps the doctor to tailor the dosage of drugs to the patient. A low red blood cell count will make the patient feel tired and breathless; a low white blood count will leave the patient with an increased risk of infection; and low platelets give the patient a higher risk of bleeding. A high blood count means the dose is probably too low and a low count that it is probably too high, so the doctor will adjust the drug dosage accordingly.

How is chemotherapy given?

Commonly, chemotherapy is given every 3 weeks, in 21-day or 28-day cycles, for anywhere from 3 months to 6 months or a year. With a 21-day cycle the drugs might be given once every 3 weeks. On a 28-day cycle they are given on day one and day eight, then there is no treatment for two weeks. The chemotherapy drugs can be given as a pill, by intravenous drip, by a combination of the two, or by injection into a vein. Some sessions last 10 minutes, some for 3 or 4 hours.

The treatment itself is not particularly painful and feels like any intravenous procedure, though sometimes the drugs cause scarring in the veins, which can make it difficult to get needles into them.

The most common combinations of drugs for breast cancer are:

- CMF (cyclophosphamide, methotrexate and 5-FU [5-fluorouracil])
- FEC (epirubicin, cyclophosphamide and 5-FU)
- E-CMF (epirubicin, followed by CMF)
- AC (doxorubicin [adriamycin] and cyclophosphamide)
- MMM (methotrexate, mitozantrone and mitomycin)
- MM (methotrexate and mitozantrone)

Doctors are investigating the relative benefits of the different combinations for different stages and types of breast cancer. Different combinations of drugs have different side effects (for instance, hair loss is more likely with FEC or AC than with CMF).

The National Epirubicin Adjuvant Trial, backed by the charity Cancer Research UK, has yielded promising results for long-term survival. The clinical trial involved more than 2000 women with early stage breast cancer from 65 hospitals across the UK and used existing drugs in a slightly different way. It compared treatment using four rounds of epirubicin followed by four rounds of standard chemotherapy (CMF) and found that, over the five years of the trial, those treated with epirubicin were 31 per cent less likely to relapse or die than women treated with the standard six rounds of CMF.

A new drug, GCSF (granulocyte colony stimulating factor), made by genetically engineering bacteria, has been found to boost the white blood cell count and hasten the bone marrow's recovery.

What determines whether or not chemotherapy is necessary?

Chemotherapy is a powerful weapon in the fight against cancer, but the doctor should explain why it is considered necessary for a particular patient and set out the benefits and side effects before a decision is made.

There are three main situations where chemotherapy is recommended: (1) before surgery (neoadjuvant chemotherapy), to shrink a large tumour and reduce the need for a mastectomy; (2) after surgery (adjuvant chemotherapy) for early stage breast cancer when the cancer has spread to the lymph nodes – radiotherapy is better for clearing up stray cancer cells in the original site, but chemotherapy is more effective when the cancer has spread to the lymph nodes and possibly beyond; (3) in advanced breast cancer, where the cancer has spread to other parts of the body, in which case the chemotherapy will be used to try and shrink the tumour, to improve symptoms, maintain a good quality of life and to prolong life where possible (see Chapter 7). It is also given instead of hormone therapy (such as tamoxifen), when the cancer cells are not hormonally sensitive (see Box 6 for a summary).

Box 6. Situations when chemotherapy is given.

- Before surgery (neoadjuvant therapy) to shrink a tumour when it is large or for inflammatory cancer.
- After surgery (adjuvant therapy), to reduce the chance that it will come back or spread.
- To control the disease when it has come back or spread to other parts of the body.
- When the cancer cells did not test positive for hormone receptors, so are unlikely to respond well to hormone therapy.
- Any combination of these.

The doctor recommends a treatment plan specific to the individual, based on things such as age, general health, type and stage of cancer, where it is located, and how much and how fast it has grown.

It is usually offered as a matter of course to women who are pre-menopausal, under the age of 50, and whose lymph nodes are positive. It is also sometimes recommended for women aged over 50 where cancer is found in the lymph nodes.

Chemotherapy drugs can stop the ovaries producing the oestrogen that can stimulate the breast tumour to grow. But the loss of oestrogen will also stop the woman's periods, either temporarily or permanently. This depends on her age and on the drugs she is given, but if periods have not restarted a year after the treatment has ended it is unlikely that the ovaries will start to work again, in which case she will be infertile.

What are some of the common short-term side effects of chemotherapy and what can be done to manage them?

There are many side effects of chemotherapy but the most common are:

- Hair loss or thinning.
- Increased risk of infection.
- Nausea and vomiting.
- Fatigue.
- Sore mouth and mouth ulcers.

The side effects depend mainly on the specific drugs and the dose and it is very important that the doctor knows about any changes in physical condition during treatment so the patient's state can be accurately assessed. Most patients do not have severe reactions to chemotherapy drugs and a few have none. Many side effects can now be controlled and most are short-term. Hair grows back within a few weeks of the treatment ending and it is often better than before. The listlessness that often accompanies chemotherapy also gradually disappears after treatment has finished.

Jill, who had an unpleasant, but short-lived side effect from her chemotherapy, says:

❝One day I thought I was going blind as well as everything else. I couldn't see the face of another Mum at the school when she called out to me from across the road. I went home crying because it felt like the last straw. I rang the chemo sister and she told me to come in and she would give me a different anti-sickness drug. Apparently, there are so many side effects to the different types of treatment that, although they list the main ones, sometimes other things happen that you don't expect and this was simply one of them. **"**

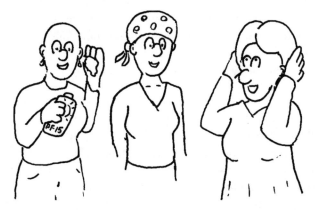

Practical ways to cope with hair loss include using a sunscreen, and wearing a turban or wig.

What can be done to ease the side effects?

Hair loss (alopecia)

Not all anti-cancer drugs cause hair loss, but many do. Sometimes the loss is hardly noticeable, but sometimes there is complete baldness and occasionally that includes the loss of eyebrows, eyelashes, leg and arm hair and pubic hair. If hair loss is going to happen it usually starts within a few weeks of starting chemotherapy, though occasionally happens almost immediately. The hair doesn't fall out all at once but comes out in large quantities overnight or when washing or brushing it.

Sometimes it is possible to use a 'cold cap' to cool the scalp and reduce the amount of chemotherapy drugs reaching the hair follicles on the head. This can reduce or even prevent hair loss, but doesn't work for everyone and is only effective with some drugs.

Kay found that the cold cap was not a solution for her. She said:

"I tried the cold cap first of all and that was horrendous – I cried while I was having that on. I'm not very good with pain – even having my legs waxed – and that was really awful. I felt as though my head was going to explode. I didn't continue with that – I think it was my Mum worrying about how I would feel about losing my hair, but I said, 'Mum, I'd rather have no hair than go through suffering the cold cap.' **"**

Many people view their hair as a very important part of their appearance and the thought of losing it can seem like the last straw. In some cultures it is a sign of fertility or status, so coming to terms with hair loss is doubly difficult.

There are some practical ways to cope, including wearing a wig, a turban or headscarf, which might make life easier during a difficult time.

But hair loss is temporary and once treatment has ended the hair will start to grow back, and sometimes it starts to come through even before treatment has ended. At first the hair is very fine, but will probably have fully grown back within 3 to 6 months:

Kay's hair grew back within 4 months:

❝My chemo finished in August and in October it was coming through again. I had a very short skinhead at Christmas time – it doesn't take too long, quite quick. It's a bit disheartening when it first comes out, though – even though I'd had my hair cut very short before the operation to make it easier for myself. It's a bit hard having a dinner party and your hair falling out, you've no control over it! When you wash it it comes out more – you're moulting, it's everywhere, all over the place.**❞**

It is sometimes curlier than before – though usually it returns to normal after a few months – and is sometimes a different colour, most commonly grey or black.

HELPFUL TIPS! HELPFUL TIPS! HELPFUL TIPS! HELPFUL

Hints for coping with hair loss

- Think about having your hair cut short before treatment starts to reduce the weight of hair on the scalp and minimise hair loss, and to give yourself time to adjust to your new appearance.
- Use baby shampoo to prevent dryness.
- Brush your hair gently, with a baby brush.
- Avoid excessive heat from hairdryers or heated rollers.
- Wear a turban or cap at night to collect loose hair.
- Avoid having perms or hair colour for at least 6 months after finishing treatment.
- Avoid nylon pillowcases, which can irritate the scalp.
- If you leave your head uncovered, use a high protection sun cream at all times.

Increased risk of infection

Patients who are receiving chemotherapy face an increased risk of infection, which means they need to take extra care in avoiding situations that might put them at risk. The chemotherapy drugs affect healthy blood cells, so patients are not only more likely to get infections but are less able to fight them.

Blood counts reach their lowest point around 10 days after injections, when fatigue and depression are likely to be at their worst.

Jill found the chemotherapy depleted her energy and spirits, but at least she avoided getting any infections. She said:

> **“**I had chemotherapy for six months and spent the time shivering and feeling miserable. A couple of times they couldn't do it because the blood count was wrong.**”**

Kay, too, found chemotherapy unpleasant:

> **“**The chemo is probably like having very bad 'flu – you can't walk, it just really turns you upside-down.**”**

Things start to improve after one chemotherapy cycle ends and are getting back to near-normal when the next cycle starts, then the blood counts slump once more, and the whole cycle starts again.

Polly's experience of chemotherapy was typical. She said:

> **“**On the day I had it I was fine for a few hours then felt absolutely terrible for a few days. All I could do was lie in bed and try not to be sick ... and generally the next morning I'd wake up feeling an awful lot better; then I'd feel not particularly well for the week, but generally at the end of the week I'd wake up and think, 'Oh, I feel quite well again,' and have a bit of an energy spurt and feel much better and generally back to normal for a couple of weeks before it all started again.**”**

Patients must seek medical help if they show signs of developing an infection while receiving chemotherapy (such as sore throat or raised temperature) as they might need urgent antibiotic treatment.

Philip was alarmed by an infection he developed during his chemotherapy. He said:

> **“**Chemo for me was fine ... but I did have one very bad scare, which probably scared me more than the actual cancer. During one of the cycles I got a chest infection which had me in hospital for a whole week because they

thought at first it was an embolism. I thought my time had come. During the chemo you have to keep taking your temperature all the time. I thought it was indigestion at first but in the morning I took my temperature, it was much higher than it normally is, so I marched straight down to the Accident and Emergency at the hospital and by the time I got there I was quite bad – really didn't know much about the first couple of days then gradually got better. My immune system just couldn't cope, so they didn't do a cycle for two or three weeks, then started after that and there were no further adventures. **"**

HELPFUL TIPS! HELPFUL TIPS! HELPFUL TIPS! HELPFUL

Hints for fighting infections

- Make sure any dental work is finished before starting chemotherapy.
- Eat a healthy diet and get plenty of rest.
- Stay away from large crowds and anyone with a cold, infection or contagious disease.
- Avoid animals, especially cat litter trays and bird cages.
- Wear gloves in the garden and the kitchen, to protect your hands against cuts and burns.

Nausea and vomiting

Nausea and vomiting – feeling sick and being sick – are common side effects of chemotherapy and the doctor can prescribe anti-emetics (drugs to prevent sickness) to help.

Kay had a novel approach to stemming the nausea, but it worked for her. She said:

"Everything they say you're going to feel, I think I felt it. I felt very sick on the first one and for the second and the rest of them I took the anti-sickness tablets and wore a wrist band with a metal thing on, like for seasickness. I don't know if it was psychological or whether it did help, but the one time I didn't put it on I felt sick – it's mind over matter. I was never actually sick, thank goodness. Just had this awful sense of smell. **"**

Some alternative techniques such as acupuncture have been found to help in controlling nausea.

Good nutrition is especially important during cancer treatment, but vitamin supplements might interact with the anti-cancer drugs, so should be avoided without medical advice.

HELPFUL TIPS! HELPFUL TIPS! HELPFUL TIPS! HELPFUL

Hints to avoid nausea

- Eat small meals often.
- Don't eat for one or two hours before treatment.
- Avoid very sweet, strong-smelling and spicy or greasy foods; instead eat bland foods such as bananas, plain rice, apples and dry toast.
- Chew your food thoroughly and eat slowly.
- Drink plenty of liquid and try sipping clear, cold water or soft drinks slowly through a straw.
- Peppermint and ginger tea might help to relieve nausea.
- Avoid caffeine and alcohol.
- Sucking ice cubes helps to freshen up the mouth.
- Acupuncture has been found to be helpful.

Fatigue

Cancer patients often feel very tired. Fatigue is a common side effect of both chemotherapy and radiotherapy and is the body's way of signalling that the body needs rest and good nutrition in its efforts to heal the damages inflicted by the cancer and the treatment. Tiredness is not constant from one day to the next and abrupt swings in energy levels are quite normal. Rest and sleep are important, but too much will make things worse.

HELPFUL TIPS! HELPFUL TIPS! HELPFUL TIPS! HELPFUL

Hints to cope with fatigue

- Eat a balanced diet, with plenty of fruits and vegetables and complex carbohydrates such as wholewheat breads.

- Conserve your energy where possible by spreading your activities throughout the day and taking frequent breaks.
- Do as much as possible while seated.
- Find activities that you enjoy that don't need much physical effort, such as listening to music or reading.
- Ask family or friends for help with household chores or childcare.

Sore mouth

Some anti-cancer drugs cause a very sore mouth and mouth ulcers. They usually start about 5 to 10 days after treatment begins and clear up within 3 or 4 weeks.

The doctor might prescribe mouthwashes to prevent infection, and most are happy to prescribe strong painkillers.

What are the possible long-term side effects?

The drugs are powerful and can have long-term side effects, some more and some less serious. They can cause a chemically induced menopause, with no periods, hot flushes and emotional mood swings. The closer to the natural menopause, the higher the risk. Women aged under 40 who receive CMF for 6 months have around 35 per cent likelihood of premature menopause and therefore infertility; for women over 40, the risk is about 90 per cent. Other drug combinations have different risk rates.

Jill, who was in her early 40 s when she was diagnosed, was distressed by the instant menopause that resulted from the chemotherapy. She said:

> ❝It was such an overnight shock – no chance of having another baby. I was 44 and I don't suppose I would have, but it was just the shock of not having that choice. I do get miserable even now, 8 years on – not sure it's anything to do with breast cancer, maybe it's getting old. Sometimes when I'm walking on my own I get quite maudlin. I say, 'Snap out of it, this won't help anyone.'❞

Chemotherapy drugs carry a small risk of chronic bone marrow suppression and second cancers, especially leukaemias.

Adriamycin is a very effective breast cancer drug but it can be toxic to the heart and could cause problems for an estimated one in 200 of those treated with it.

Summary

- Chemotherapy drugs kill or damage cancer cells, either in the original tumour or where they have spread elsewhere in the body.

- They kill rapidly dividing cancer cells and therefore the cancer, but also rapidly dividing normal cells such as hair, digestive track and bone marrow cells, which is why they can cause extensive side effects.

- Blood counts are taken before and during treatment to help the doctors adjust drug dosage to the patient.

- Chemotherapy is given: before surgery, to shrink the tumour; after surgery for early stage breast cancer, particularly where it has spread to the lymph nodes; in more advanced disease, where the cancer has spread elsewhere in the body; where the cancer cells are not hormonally responsive.

- The most common short-term side effects are: hair loss or thinning; increased risk of infection; nausea and vomiting; fatigue; and sore mouth.

- The most common long-term side effect is premature menopause, but there is a small risk of chronic bone marrow suppression and second cancers or of heart problems, particularly with some of the drugs.

Hormonal therapies and immunotherapy

12

Overview

It has been known for more than 100 years that reducing the level of the female hormone oestrogen could make some breast cancers shrink. More recently it has been discovered that most of the ones that shrink contain oestrogen receptors. Hormonal therapies are used for women with this type of tumour. This chapter looks at when hormonal therapies are used and examines two of the best known – tamoxifen and anastrozole (Arimidex) – and their possible side effects. It also considers the benefit of removing or de-activating the ovaries and the use of immunotherapy (sometimes called biological therapy) and herceptin.

What are hormonal therapies and who benefits from them?

Hormonal therapies are used to treat women whose tumour cells have been tested and found to depend for their growth on the female hormones oestrogen or progesterone (see Chapter 7, p. 52). If the cells are responsive to hormones, any cancer cells left behind after surgery or radiotherapy may continue to grow when these hormones are present in the body.

Hormonal therapy can be used to treat breast cancer before or after surgery, but is more commonly used once the tumour has been removed, to starve any remaining cancer cells and prevent the cancer returning. The ovaries, which are the source of the oestrogen in pre-menopausal women, can also be switched off by surgically removing them or treating them with drugs. This can be an important treatment for metastatic disease in women with an oestrogen receptor positive tumour.

Goserelin (Zoladex) is a type of hormonal therapy that is given to pre-menopausal women as a monthly injection to shut down the ovaries temporarily. It can be used in an effort to protect them while chemotherapy is in progress or to shrink the tumour or slow down its rate of growth. Once treatment has ended it is hoped the ovaries will start to work again, so the patient will not become permanently infertile. A study published in the *European Journal of Cancer* in August 2003 (Kaufmann *et al.*, 2003) indicates that goserelin is a promising new drug, and an effective alternative to CMF chemotherapy as adjuvant therapy for pre-menopausal women with oestrogen-positive, node-positive early breast cancer.

There is no evidence that hormonal therapies will reduce the risk of recurrence or increase the survival rate if the tumour is not sensitive to oestrogen. This does not mean that women whose cancer is node-negative have a worse prognosis, it does mean that the treatment will be different.

Tamoxifen

Tamoxifen is the best-known and most widely prescribed hormonal therapy for early- and advanced-stage breast cancer and has been used successfully for more than 25 years. The way it works is complicated and not yet fully understood, but its main effect is to block oestrogen to the breast, while acting like oestrogen in other organs.

Tamoxifen (which is also manufactured under different brand names) is taken as a tablet once a day. It can be used alone or after chemotherapy for pre- or post-menopausal women. When women with oestrogen-positive breast cancer take tamoxifen they not only cut the risk of the original cancer recurring, but also reduce the risk of developing a cancer in the other breast by 30 to 50 per cent (e.g. someone with a 10 per cent risk would reduce that to 7 or 5 per cent).

Tamoxifen is usually prescribed for 5 years, and 20 mg is the standard dose. There is some evidence that users can become resistant to tamoxifen if they take it for longer than five years and that taking it for longer might actually harm them. It is most commonly prescribed for women who are oestrogen-positive and might also help if the breast cancer cells are progesterone-positive.

As well as its benefits in fighting cancer, tamoxifen also lowers cholesterol and slows osteoporosis, which is particularly important for post-menopausal women. And, unlike chemotherapy, it does not push pre-menopausal women into the menopause.

Many women have no side effects from taking tamoxifen, and some have fewer with one brand than another, but the commonest side effects are:

- Hot flushes and night sweats which sometimes lessen over the first few months, but often continue for as long as tamoxifen is taken. Cutting down on tea, coffee, nicotine and alcohol sometimes helps and acupuncture has been found to be effective in reducing them.

- Nausea and indigestion – taking tamoxifen with food or milk at night can relieve nausea.
- Weight gain.
- Vaginal discharge or vaginal dryness.
- Blurry vision and, occasionally, cataracts.

Jill, who was 44 and still menstruating when she started chemotherapy and tamoxifen, went into a sudden and early menopause with unpleasant hot flushes as a result of her treatment. She said:

> **"**I can remember standing in the building society queue and having a really bad hot flush creep up my neck and over my whole body. I felt like I was swelling up and itchy and turning red. I shed my anorak, then my jumper and was pulling at my T-shirt neck when it was my turn!**"**

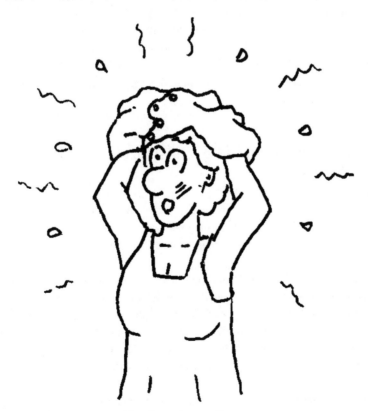

Hot flushes are a common side effect of tamoxifen.

Doctors stress that the benefits of tamoxifen far outweigh the risks for women who have already been diagnosed with breast cancer because it treats the cancer already there and halves the chance of getting cancer in the other breast. But serious side effects – while rare – have been reported and should be weighed against the proven benefits. These include a slightly greater risk of developing cancer of the uterus – which does not apply to women who have had a hysterectomy. The women most at risk, according to an American study (Bernstein *et al.*, 1999), appear to be those who in the past have taken oestrogen replacement therapy on its own and without added progestin. The risk of uterine cancer is still very small, and the majority of these cancers can be cured by hysterectomy, but it is important that if there is any abnormal bleeding it is reported immediately to the doctor.

In a few patients who take tamoxifen in combination with chemotherapy, some have reported blood clots, which can result in strokes, heart attacks, or death. Other risks include pulmonary embolism and deep vein thrombosis, especially in the legs.

Younger women taking tamoxifen might become pregnant more easily and should use an effective barrier contraceptive to prevent it because the drug can damage the foetus.

Women who have serious concerns about the possible side effects of tamoxifen should discuss them with their doctor. And anyone who does not have breast cancer but is at high risk of developing it and is considering taking tamoxifen as a prophylactic (a preventive) should talk to their doctor about the risks related to their own circumstances.

Aromatase inhibitors (e.g. anastrozole, brand name Arimidex)

Other drugs called aromatase inhibitors are an alternative to tamoxifen as hormonal therapy. Women who are past their menopause no longer produce oestrogen from their ovaries, but still produce a small amount from their adrenal glands via an enzyme called aromatase.

The process by which it is produced is called aromatisation so the drugs that block that process are called aromatase inhibitors. Anastrozole (Arimidex) is a man-made drug that prevents the production of this oestrogen, so it is most often used with post-menopausal women. It is most commonly prescribed for those whose breast cancer has spread, but recent trials with anastrozole suggest it could usefully be extended to post-menopausal women with oestrogen-positive early breast cancer.

The research shows it is more effective than tamoxifen, has fewer side effects and fewer safety concerns with long-term use. It also appears to reduce the chance of a woman developing endometrial cancer and dangerous blood clots. Like tamoxifen, it is taken as a tablet once a day and, like that drug, can cause hot flushes and nausea. But unlike tamoxifen it is known to deplete bone density and increase the risk of broken bones. And there are also some concerns that stopping the production of oestrogen altogether could adversely affect other things, such as cognitive function.

Other ways of switching off oestrogen production

Another way to switch off the supply of hormones at source for pre-menopausal women is by surgically removing or chemically de-activating the ovaries. Surgical removal (oophorectomy), unfortunately, is irreversible and there is no guarantee before the operation that it will work in halting the cancer.

There are some drugs that will induce a temporary menopause. One that was originally developed for endometriosis and has been tested for breast cancer is goserelin (also known as Zoladex). There are others, known as pituitary down-regulators (LH-RH analogues) that are given by monthly injection to temporarily stop the ovaries working in pre-menopausal women. Women who are close to the menopause when they start treatment may find their ovaries do not start again when they stop taking the drug. These drugs decrease bone density, so should only be used for a short period of time.

Immunotherapy (biological therapy)

Immunotherapy (sometimes called biological therapy) uses the body's immune system, either directly or indirectly, to fight cancer or lessen the side effects of cancer treatments.

Cancer might develop when the immune system breaks down and immunotherapies are designed to repair, stimulate or enhance its responses.

Herceptin (trastuzumab) belongs to a new group of cancer drugs called monoclonal antibodies (MOAB). It provides a treatment for the one in five patients with advanced breast cancers that have spread, and whose tumours produce excess amounts of a protein known as HER-2. Herceptin works by interfering with one of the ways in which breast cancer cells divide and grow and by enhancing the body's own immune response. HER-2 is a growth factor receptor which transmits signals from outside the cancer cell to the inside, and makes the cells grow. Herceptin, the antibody, attaches itself to this protein, thus stopping the cells from dividing and growing. It also appears to increase the effect of chemotherapy drugs on breast cancer and could help women who have not responded to chemotherapy on its own.

Herceptin is given as an infusion into a vein once a week. The treatment takes about an hour and appears to have few severe side effects, although it can cause serious allergic reactions and damage to the heart. It is still a relatively new treatment but appears to be promising.

Summary

- Hormonal therapies are a systemic treatment used for women with tumours that have been tested and found to depend for their growth on the female hormones oestrogen or progesterone.

- Hormonal therapies can be used before or after surgery but are usually used after the cancer has been removed to reduce the risk of it returning.

- Tamoxifen, the best-known and most widely prescribed hormonal therapy, works by blocking oestrogen to the breast, while acting like oestrogen in other organs.

- Tamoxifen commonly causes hot flushes and sometimes other minor side effects, but occasionally there are more serious side effects such as an increased risk of uterine cancer.

- Aromatase inhibitors such as anastrozole (Arimidex) block the production of oestrogen by the adrenal gland, which is the main source of the hormone in post-menopausal women, and have been shown to be even more effective than tamoxifen in cutting the risk of cancer recurring in oestrogen-positive cancers.

- The ovaries of pre-menopausal women (particularly with cancer that has metastasised) are sometimes surgically removed or chemically de-activated to cut the production of oestrogen to cancer cells.

- Immunotherapy (or biological therapy) uses the body's immune system, either directly or indirectly, to fight cancer or lessen the side effects of cancer treatments.

- Herceptin (trastuzumab) belongs to a new group of cancer drugs called monoclonal antibodies and is used to treat patients with advanced breast cancers that have spread, and whose tumours produce excess protein HER-2.

Breast cancer, pregnancy and fertility

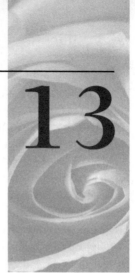

13

Overview

Because many women are delaying pregnancy until they are in their 30s and early 40s, increasing numbers of women are pregnant when they find they have breast cancer. And others, having delayed their pregnancy, want to know if they face extra risks if they have been treated for breast cancer and then become pregnant. Both groups are usually concerned about the likely long-term impact of treatment on their fertility. This chapter examines the treatment options for a woman who is pregnant or breastfeeding when she is diagnosed with breast cancer. It also looks at some of the risks of pregnancy after breast cancer and the effects of treatment on fertility.

Diagnosis during pregnancy

Diagnosis is not always easy, because the changes in a woman's breast that happen in pregnancy mask the signals that would normally alert her to the possibility of cancer. And some of the standard diagnostic tools, such as mammogram, are avoided for fear of damaging the baby.

It is as important for the woman to be aware of the way her breast normally feels during pregnancy, as it is at any other time. Breast cancer in pregnancy is rare, but it does happen, so any suspicious lump should be investigated then, as it would be at any other time. A biopsy, if necessary, is best done under local anaesthesia to avoid exposing the foetus to general anaesthesia.

For a woman who is already pregnant when breast cancer is diagnosed, there are some difficult decisions. The stage of the foetus and the stage of the cancer will determine what can be offered. She could opt for termination to permit more aggressive treatment – depending on her views on abortion and on how much that particular pregnancy means to her. Or she could choose to keep the child and tailor the treatment to fit in with her pregnancy. This might mean accepting that some of the more effective treatments are not available until after her child is born.

If she has an early stage cancer (Stage I or II) and is in the first 3 months of pregnancy (the first trimester), the doctor would probably recommend a biopsy followed by wide excision under local anaesthetic because of the dangers of a general anaesthetic to the foetus. If it turns out that a mastectomy and chemotherapy are needed this could be given in the second (i.e. 3 to 6 months) or third trimester (6 to 9 months), but radiation therapy, which is harmful to the unborn child at any stage of development, would be delayed until after it was born.

A woman with advanced cancer has an even more difficult choice. She can choose to delay treatment until the first 3 months have passed, then have chemotherapy which is not aggressive enough to harm the baby, but might be less damaging to the cancer. She can delay treatment until after the baby is born, which might put her own life at risk. Or she could choose to have an abortion, knowing that the anti-cancer drugs might damage her ovaries and make her infertile. There is no evidence that having an abortion improves the prognosis, but it makes treatment easier. Whatever the decision, she will need plenty of emotional support. But it is her decision.

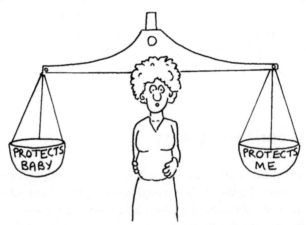

There are difficult decisions for women who are pregnant when breast cancer is diagnosed.

What about breastfeeding after treatment ends?

A woman who is diagnosed during pregnancy or immediately afterwards would have to wean the baby on to a bottle once she started chemotherapy as the drugs would pass into the breast milk and harm the child.

But the possibility of her future ability to breastfeed after cancer treatment depends on the extent of the tumour and the treatment chosen. Smaller, early-stage tumours are more likely to leave the woman with the structures she needs for breastfeeding than the larger, later-stage tumours. Radiotherapy could permanently damage the lobules and ducts in the affected breast, but the unaffected breast could still be used for breastfeeding.

Risks of recurrence following treatment for breast cancer

Becoming pregnant after having breast cancer will not make the cancer spread, but no one knows whether it will make any microscopic cells left behind grow faster. If the cancer was very aggressive, a lot of lymph nodes were positive, or there was some other factor that increased the risk of micrometastases, these risks might be included in the decision about whether to try for a baby.

Fertility and treatment

Chemotherapy can cause an early menopause, which of course means the woman will be infertile. The closer she is to the natural menopause when treatment starts, the higher the risk that the chemicals will stop her periods permanently. The average age of menopause is 51 and the risk of chemotherapy-induced menopause for a woman of 45 is 80 to 90 per cent but 15 to 20 per cent for a 35-year-old, depending on the drugs used.

It is difficult to be sure which women will become post-menopausal as a result of the chemotherapy, but it is important to consider this as a possibility before treatment starts. And when making a decision it is a good idea to be entirely clear about how important the chemotherapy is in preventing recurrence. If the doctor says that chemotherapy will halve the chance of the cancer coming back it sounds pretty convincing. But if the risk of recurrence is only 4 or 5 per cent, that means the chemotherapy reduces the risk to 2 or 2.5 per cent, and the difference in risk might not warrant the price for some women.

Kay was 31 when she was diagnosed with Stage I/II cancer and coped well with the mastectomy, chemotherapy and radiotherapy that followed. But she found the thought of becoming infertile because of her treatment very distressing. She said :

❝I think the only time I got a bit depressed was at Christmas and that was after seeing the plastic surgeon about my reconstruction, who said I couldn't have children afterwards. But I've been on the internet and my breast surgeon said you can. I think they were just covering themselves because they think you might be infertile with the chemotherapy. **"**

Fertility drugs

No one knows how safe the fertility drugs are that are used for in vitro fertilisation (IVF) or for boosting ovulation, or how they relate to breast cancer. But other hormones such as DES (diethylstilbestrol), prescribed from the 1940s to the 1960s to boost fertility, prevent miscarriage or inhibit milk production, and those used in hormone replacement therapy (HRT), have been shown to increase the risk of breast cancer, so it seems likely that fertility drugs also do.

Polly, a trainee anesthetist married to a GP, was 30 when she was diagnosed with a Grade 3 ductal carcinoma. She and her husband want to have children, but recognise that storing eggs prior to treatment is a risky business as the hormones that are used to stimulate the ovaries could also stimulate the tumour and encourage it to grow. Polly said:

> **"**I went on to Zoladex, a new drug which gave me a temporary menopause, because we haven't had children yet and because of the likelihood of the chemotherapy affecting my ovaries. I went to see a fertility person and she said there's not a lot they can do because my tumour receptors were strongly oestrogen-positive and they didn't want to give me stimulating hormones before the chemotherapy to collect the eggs.
>
> They said there's this bit of experimental work – perhaps if you shut down your ovaries as you start the chemotherapy it might not affect them quite as much. I thought it makes sense to have a bit of time shutting everything down and I'm on tamoxifen as well. **"**

Saving embryos

Some women who are at risk of premature menopause consider having their eggs preserved before treatment starts, so they can have children later. But although egg collection and freezing is being done, as is ovarian tissue collection, it is still relatively experimental. Eggs, where they are preserved, have normally been fertilised, which means the woman must have a sperm donor or partner before her embryos can be stored. A recent court case, in which the woman's partner vetoed the embryos' continued existence, highlights the possible complications. A further problem arises from the need to give the woman high doses of hormones to stimulate the eggs' growth so they can be harvested, which is a risky strategy when she is being treated for breast cancer. Another problem is that egg collection takes time and will usually delay treatment.

Summary

- Breast cancer is rare during pregnancy but does happen and diagnosis is difficult because the breast changes that result from pregnancy can mask the signs of cancer.

- The stage of the foetus and the stage of the cancer will determine what treatment is offered, but the doctor would recommend delaying mastectomy and chemotherapy until the second or third trimester and radiotherapy and/or hormonal therapy until after the baby was born.

- Before chemotherapy is started after the baby's birth the woman will have to wean the baby on to a bottle, because the drugs would pass into the breast milk and harm the child.

- Future ability to breastfeed after cancer treatment depends on the extent of the tumour and the treatment.

- Becoming pregnant will not make the cancer spread, but could make any microscopic cells left behind grow faster.

- Chemotherapy can cause early menopause and therefore infertility, though the chances are increased for those closest to the age of the natural menopause and it is difficult to predict who will be affected.

- No one knows how safe fertility drugs are, but it seems likely they have some effect on breast cancer.

- Egg collection and freezing is still at an experimental stage and a woman's eggs are usually fertilised before they can be stored; she must have high doses of hormones before they are harvested and egg collection will delay treatment.

How does it feel to live with breast cancer?

14

Overview

After breast cancer has been diagnosed and the treatment is over, life goes on. But it is never quite the same as it was before the diagnosis. This chapter looks at some of the changes that face women after surgery and chemotherapy. It also describes some ways you can protect yourself from the cancer's recurrence and possibly from getting it in the first place.

What are the changes after treatment?

A diagnosis of cancer must rank as one of the most stressful events in anyone's life. For some, the outlook is much more hopeful than for others, but initially just about everyone thinks they are going to die. Once treatment gets under way – no matter how unpleasant – things seem to be better because you are doing something to get rid of the cancer and the situation is eased by the care of healthcare professionals and the solicitude of family and friends for the lucky ones. Some people feel – in among all the upset – a sort of guilty thrill that they are centre stage in something important and dramatic. But once the drama of diagnosis and treatment are finished and the patients are left to get on with their lives without the support of the rest of the cast, it can feel as though they have been pushed out into a bleak, cold place. One issue they often have to face, after surgery for breast cancer, is a change in the way they think about their body and the effect that that has on their sexual feelings and sexual activity.

Body image and the effect on sex

Getting used to a new body image is particularly difficult when the change is linked to deeply held beliefs about yourself and who you are. Women value their breasts as an indication of their femininity and sexuality, as well as an important and emotionally powerful means of nurturing their babies. Meanwhile, the tabloids present an endless stream of photographs of women flaunting their bodies, with stories and conjectures about women who have had, or might have had, breast enhancement operations. It is unsurprising that the loss of a breast is seen by many as a major blow, and that women sometimes have problems in shifting the focus of their self-value.

It is misguided to generalise about people's emotional response to surgery and to assume that their distress diminishes with age. Many elderly women are very upset by the loss of a breast and the change in their body image – having lost one marker of their femininity with the menopause, this is seen as yet another blow.

Molly (diagnosed at 62, now aged 76) had a lumpectomy, but still found it difficult to come to terms with the way her body looked after surgery. She said:

> ❝I've never really acknowledged it or worked it through, but I don't think I've ever felt the same about my body – the fact that my right breast has been spoiled because it's a slightly funny shape and where it was cut – right on the top – it bulges a bit over the cut. By the time you get to my age everything's sagged anyway, so what the hell, but you mourn the fact that your body's not what it used to be.❞

It should not be assumed, either, that the older woman is not a sexual being, and is not affected by the change in body image and its possible impact on her sex life. The loss of a breast can be difficult for a woman of any age and for her long-term partner, and changes in their relationship can inhibit sexual activity for psychological reasons. Sometimes the man refrains from sexual contact because of his concern for his partner's well-being. She, however, takes it as a rejection and feels even more unattractive. Then neither wants to make the first move. Sometimes, too, the change from being two equal, healthy partners to being patient and carer can inhibit the expression of sexual feelings. Chemotherapy can bring on an early menopause, and this too – combined with the other issues around breast cancer – can severely affect a woman's libido, whether because of its psychological effect or its effect on her hormones.

Given time, most (though not all) partners are able to adapt to the patient's changed body and the patient's libido returns to normal. Sometimes, however, it is a good idea to seek help from professional counsellors, before any frustrations and misunderstandings become entrenched.

Jill, aged 44 when she had her mastectomy, 8 years ago, is still trying to come to terms with her mastectomy and is still affected by her feelings about it. Her husband is loving but avoids touching it. She said:

> **❝**My husband never touches my mutilated side. It is pretty horrid – bony and lumpy. You can feel the ribs and the folds in the scar tissue. But I wish he would touch it sometimes, because it's my body now and I can still feel it. I wonder if it's similar – although nowhere near as bad – as having a foot cut off, because I can sometimes feel my nipple itch, only to realise that it's my prosthesis side that's itching. Our sex life is fine really. We're an old married couple and I feel loved and cosy, but if I was single I am conscious that it's very unattractive to have one huge breast and absolutely nothing on the other side. I would want to keep my bra and prosthesis on if I was with someone new.**❞**

Some women feel unable to explore new relationships, while others go off the rails for a while, to reassure themselves that they are still attractive.

Kay, who is 34 now, had her mastectomy two days after her 32nd birthday and set out to prove to herself that she was still desirable. She said:

> **❝**I've probably been more promiscuous than I ever was before. The first time was when I was on holiday and they knew, because they could see in my bikini I didn't have a bosom, but I've had no bad reactions ... [he] was very, very young and he just made me feel really good and it's something I did just to get past that first stage, I suppose. I've had no terrible reactions to it.**❞**

Because of its rarity, men can feel particularly isolated. Just as women can feel that their sexual identity is assailed by the treatment for breast cancer, it is often assumed that men might feel their masculinity is threatened by suffering from a disease that is predominantly experienced by women, and one that is related to hormone imbalances. Yet this is not necessarily borne out by research. One ongoing study at Cardiff University (Iredale, 2003) has so far found little evidence for widespread embarrassment at the diagnosis, though it has found that many men were not aware before their own experience that breast cancer could also affect them.

Philip, aged 40 when he was diagnosed in March 2000, has no problem about body image, saying 'it's almost like a badge of honour'. He believes, however, that men need to be more aware that they, too, can get breast cancer:

> **❝**It was a total surprise that men could get it. My partner had had a couple of cysts and I'd said, 'Look, there's a bloke going into one of the cubicles,'

and she said, 'Well, blokes get cancer as well.' I don't think it had really sunk in, but obviously I found out that they do. I don't see it as a female ailment – I do get slightly annoyed when I hear about it and they never mention that blokes get it as well. I think if the awareness was a little bit higher then blokes might look into if they feel a lump. My partner said, 'You ought to get that checked out.' If I'd been by myself I don't know whether I'd have gone that quickly. **"**

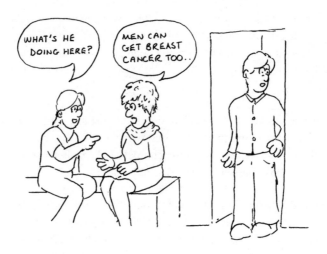

How can you protect yourself from recurrence?

Given that there is no incontrovertible cause for breast cancer, there is no sure way you can protect yourself from developing it or from stopping its recurrence. Nevertheless, there are some clues. Researchers are increasingly convinced of the importance of diet and are investigating the dietary habits of women in those countries where there is a low incidence of breast cancer. There is evidence that eating a diet that is rich in fruit and vegetables may give some protection from breast cancer, while a diet that is high in red or processed meat (such as sausages, burgers and pies) may increase the risks. And studies in Norway and America have shown that women who exercise and are consistently active have a decreased risk of breast cancer.

Evidence suggests the following measures might help to cut the risk of breast cancer:

- Take lots of exercise.
- Breastfeed your baby for longer.

- Eat lots of fresh fruit and vegetables and plenty of fibre.
- Take a daily multi-vitamin/mineral supplement, especially the anti-oxidant vitamins A, C and E and selenium (but don't overdo it – large doses of vitamin A can be damaging and too much selenium can be toxic).
- Cut down on alcohol consumption (the burden it places on your liver means it is less able to deal with the oestrogen).
- If you drink more than one glass of wine a day, folate supplements (vitamin Bc, or the synthetic form of folate known as folic acid) of 400 mcg daily are believed to give some protection (it's found in beetroots, green leafy vegetables such as brussel sprouts, and wholegrain foods, but foods alone are unlikely to provide enough).

Preventive (prophylactic) mastectomy

Some women are so terrified of the possibility of breast cancer that they have both breasts removed. Their fears are usually based on finding that they, or a close female relative, have a faulty gene – BRCA1 or BRCA2 – which will significantly increase the likelihood of developing breast cancer. Even this drastic step is not a foolproof way of heading off the disease, as there is no way to guarantee that all the breast tissue will be removed, but there is research that supports the belief that having a double mastectomy greatly reduces the risk.

Tamoxifen or anastrozole (brand name Arimidex) used as preventives

Tamoxifen (an anti-oestrogen, see Chapter 12) is a complicated drug: it blocks oestrogen in some organs, but acts like oestrogen in others. As it blocks oestrogen to the breast, it reduces the risk of recurrence of the original cancer and also reduces the risk of cancer occurring in the opposite breast by 30 to 50 per cent. Some studies have shown that women who are at high risk of breast cancer but have not yet developed it can cut the risk considerably by taking tamoxifen. Others have not found it makes much difference, but the studies are ongoing. And tamoxifen will only work on those tumours that are sensitive to hormones.

There are also risks from taking tamoxifen – of endometrial cancer, stroke, pulmonary embolism and deep vein thrombosis – and these increase after the age of 50. It could be that some women will die from a heart attack caused by the drugs to cure a cancer they might never have had.

Anastrozole (an aromatase inhibitor, see Chapter 12), in a study coordinated by Cancer Research UK (Cuzick *et al.*, 2003), has recently been found to be even more effective than tamoxifen in reducing the risk of breast cancer recurrence, and researchers are currently investigating whether it will be as effective in preventing the disease as in treating it. It blocks the production of oestrogen in post-menopausal women and has fewer side effects than tamoxifen, but women taking anastrozole are more likely to suffer osteoporosis.

Summary

- Many women and their partners have problems adjusting to the changed body image after surgery for breast cancer and this can cause sexual problems which might need help from professional counsellors.

- Men are often assumed to feel their sexual identity is threatened by suffering from a disease predominantly experienced by women, but this is not necessarily the case.

- There is no clear cause for breast cancer, so there is no certain way to prevent it, but research suggests that eating lots of fruit and vegetables, restricting alcohol consumption and taking plenty of exercise is helpful.

- There is some evidence that women at high risk of breast cancer because they have the BRCA1 or BRCA2 genes will significantly cut their risk if they have both breasts removed.

- Tamoxifen and anastrazole are both useful in reducing the risk of breast cancer recurring and are being tested for their use as preventives.

Complementary therapies, holistic practice and diet

Overview

Complementary therapies are increasingly popular as a way of supplementing conventional treatment, and growing numbers of doctors are beginning to offer them as valuable extras. This chapter looks at the meaning of 'complementary' and 'alternative' therapies and the underlying holistic principle. It looks at the reasons why people use them and some of the different therapies that are classed as 'complementary'. It looks briefly at the work of the Bristol Cancer Help Centre, then outlines the methods, aims and possible side effects of the different complementary therapies. It concludes with a look at alternative therapies and the effect of diet on cancer.

What is complementary therapy?

Some people talk about 'complementary' and 'alternative' therapies as though they mean the same thing, but complementary therapies are designed to supplement mainstream medicine, while alternative therapies are intended to replace it. Complementary and alternative therapies are not currently in standard use because most have not yet been subjected to rigorous scientific scrutiny. However, many doctors are becoming more open to the idea that their 'holistic' principles have something to commend them and are beginning to offer some of the complementary therapies alongside regular NHS cancer treatments such as surgery, radiotherapy and chemotherapy. Alternative therapies generally involve special diets, extra vitamins and herbal medicine and are mostly based on boosting the immune system to a level where it can fight off the cancer. They remain – until subjected to proper research – a very risky option.

Holistic practice and many complementary therapies are based on an underlying belief that health depends on the harmonious co-existence of body, emotions, mind and spirit: illness happens when there is an imbalance between the different elements, or a blockage of energy in any part of the system. Although some of the holistic theories about illness seem a long way from those of traditional medicine, they don't seem so different if you think in terms of taking account of physical, psychological, emotional and spiritual factors to find effective treatments for the individual. They are used mainly to alleviate physical side effects and enhance the patient's quality of life and, whether or not you accept the rationale behind complementary therapies, many of them do seem to work. There are other holistic theories, which seem to imply that the illness is the patient's fault or is a punishment, that are inappropriate and potentially damaging.

People with breast cancer use complementary therapies for different reasons. Some do so because they feel that the conventional medical process is out of their hands and that using complementary treatments gives back some control over their healing. Others turn to them to improve their quality of life by reducing the side effects of chemotherapy. And still others find that complementary therapies give them more hope that they will survive.

Many complementary therapies have been shown to be very valuable in improving people's quality of life by enhancing their mental health, reducing pain and alleviating the side effects of regular cancer regimes. But, while most are not harmful, when administered by unqualified practitioners some have the potential for inflicting injury or for dangerous interactions with conventional treatment. Most complementary therapies are not regulated by law, but usually have a professional body and recognised qualifications to practise safely. It is important that patients should check with their doctor before using these therapies as some can interact with chemotherapy or other prescription drugs.

There are many different therapies that are classed as 'complementary' but the ones most commonly used for breast cancer are: acupuncture (and acupressure), aromatherapy, creative therapies, herbal medicine, homeopathy, hypnotherapy, relaxation and visualisation, and reflexology. NHS patients who would like complementary therapy need to be referred by their doctor, usually their GP.

What is the Bristol Cancer Help Centre?

The Bristol Cancer Help Centre is one of the best-known venues in the UK where complementary therapies are practised. It was founded in 1980 by acupuncturist Penny Brohn, and her friend, Pat Pilkington, following Penny's diagnosis with breast cancer the previous year. The Centre's aim is to provide a holistic approach and a place where 'body, mind and spirit could be thought about simultaneously' but under strong medical guidance.

Six television programmes, called *A Gentle Way with Cancer*, broadcast in 1983, fuelled the original small Centre's growth and later that year a new, much bigger centre was opened by the Prince of Wales. Then, in 1990, the Centre became the centre of adverse publicity resulting from research which the Charities Commission condemned as 'fatally flawed' and inadequately supervised. It has been gradually rebuilding its credibility since then, and growing numbers of people are convinced of the benefits of its holistic approach to physical, emotional and spiritual well-being.

Trish, who was 42 when she was diagnosed, was 'completely numb, really very, very shocked' by the news that she had breast cancer. After a lumpectomy the doctors recommended chemotherapy, radiotherapy and tamoxifen, but she felt frightened and went to the Bristol Cancer Help Centre to sort out her feelings. She said:

> ❝When I got there I was in complete turmoil and confusion and I felt – I'll have a week here, if nothing happens at least I've got a week out – I can rest and not have to answer to anybody, friends or family, I can just sit and think about what happens next.
>
> It was honestly life-changing, it really was. I learnt so much about myself and how to deal with – life, really. It's tragic that you have to get cancer to go there, because everyone would benefit from knowing how to deal with problems.❞

After leaving Bristol, Trish decided to have radiotherapy, but she used the visualisation techniques she had learnt there to cope with the treatment.

The Centre's two main aims are: to help people with cancer and their carers to deal with the diagnosis and treatment; and to help promote their health by empowering them and encouraging them to develop a 'nurturing, responsible and protective relationship' with themselves.

That is also the aim of those health professionals in the NHS who choose to offer complementary therapies. The following are some that are used in the Bristol Cancer Centre and elsewhere.

Acupuncture

Acupuncture is one of the few complementary therapies that has been subjected to proper scientific testing and, although there is no evidence that it can affect the cancer itself, there is convincing evidence that it can reduce some of the more common side effects of treatment, such as nausea, vomiting and hot flushes.

According to traditional Chinese medical theory, the energy-flow (*qi*), which governs health, travels around the body along 'meridians'. When this flow is disrupted, the theory goes, disease can happen. Acupuncture is the practice of inserting very fine needles into specific points along the meridians where the imbalances of energy can be corrected. A Westernised view of this suggests that acupuncture influences neurotransmitters and endorphins, which are chemicals and hormones in the body that can alleviate pain.

Acupuncture is regarded as safe when administered by a properly qualified practitioner, but serious side effects can arise if the practitioner is not well trained. Acupuncture is not advised for people with low platelet counts or those on anticoagulants (blood-thinning drugs) as it can cause bleeding.

Acupressure and electroacupuncture

Acupressure is based on the same theory as acupuncture but instead of using needles the energy points are stimulated by pressure from the fingertips.

Electroacupuncture is another variation and uses electrical impulses to stimulate the energy points – either directly or through acupuncture needles.

Neither therapy has been as well studied as acupuncture, but there is evidence that they can help to reduce nausea and possibly stress. Patients should discuss the possible side effects with their doctor before undergoing treatment.

Aromatherapy

Aromatherapists believe that the highly concentrated essential oils extracted from flowers, fruit, seeds, leaves and the bark of trees, have healing properties. They usually use the oil for massage (though it must be diluted in a carrier oil such as grapeseed or sweet almond before being applied to the skin) but they also use them for inhalations, in baths or as a cold compress.

Aromatherapy is used to alleviate specific symptoms or to relieve pain or stress.

There are concerns about the possible interaction of the oils with the drugs used in chemotherapy, so it is important to check with the doctor before treatment and to consult a qualified practitioner.

Creative therapies

Creative therapies – including music and art therapies – are widely used in many palliative care units and some other mainstream healthcare settings both during and after treatment. They are believed to bypass the conscious brain and tap into the subconscious, thereby releasing emotions or insights. Trained art therapists can help patients with no previous training in either music or art to express emotions they find difficult to express in words.

Herbal medicine

Herbal medicine is a system that uses various remedies derived from plants and plant extracts – including the stems, leaves and flowers of herbaceous plants, the bark of trees and rhizomes, roots and bulbs. Plants and herbs have been an important source of medicinal remedies for thousands of years and many traditional drugs, such as aspirin, are derived from plants. Herbal remedies usually contain more than one active ingredient, but pharmaceutical companies generally produce their drugs by isolating just the substance that seems to make the herb effective. There are dozens of herbs that are promoted as helpful for breast cancer – including aloe vera, burdock, Echinacea, Essiac, a herbal tea, green tea, milk thistle and red clover – and an increasing number of research studies are investigating their effects. So far, however, most have not been tested under rigorous scientific conditions, so it is impossible to vouch for their effectiveness or safety. It is important to check with the doctor before using herbal remedies, in case there are interactions with chemotherapy drugs.

Trish visited a Chinese herbalist who prescribed a combination of herbs that she is convinced alleviated her radiotherapy symptoms. She said:

> **❝**I noticed a huge difference very quickly. I was being very sick and very tired and very depressed with it, but within two or three days I felt much better and better able to cope.**❞**

Homeopathy

Homeopathy is thought to work on the immune system and is based on the 'law of similars', the theory that 'like cures like': highly diluted doses of drugs that would produce symptoms like those of the illness being treated are administered to promote self-healing.

The homeopath will take the patient's overall health history before deciding which homeopathic remedies to recommend. Medical opinion is divided about the value of homeopathy, but some NHS hospitals offer it to alleviate some of the side effects of radiotherapy or chemotherapy. Again, the patient should consult her doctor before taking these remedies.

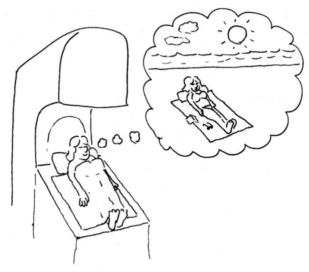

There is some evidence that visualisation can help reduce pain and uncomfortable side effects.

Hypnotherapy, relaxation and visualisation

Hypnotherapists usually begin their sessions with relaxation exercises to encourage patients to reach an extreme state of relaxation – a trance-like state – where they can communicate directly with the subconscious mind.

They see the subconscious as 'the powerhouse' that drives emotions, and aim to break down habits of thinking that reside there and contribute to anxiety. They do this by using visualisation techniques, which are based on the belief that you can make virtually anything happen if you can create a strong enough mental image of it happening, while affirming to yourself that you can and will make it come about.

Visualisation images used in this way should picture the body's defences as powerful and effective and the cancer cells as weak and vulnerable. They can include representations such as soldiers killing the cancer cells or sharks eating them. The images are usually accompanied by silent or spoken affirmations, 'ego-strengthening' statements affirming one's self-worth and intentions to achieve health and become free of pain. It is important to phrase the statements positively rather than negatively, for instance 'I am growing healthier every day', rather than 'I will not feel sick today' which focuses the mind on sickness; and in the present, rather than the future, for example 'I am healthy', not 'I will be healthy'.

There is some sound evidence that visualisation combined with medication can reduce pain and uncomfortable side effects of cancer treatments, and anecdotal evidence of more dramatic effects. And whether or not it contributes to healing, it gives those who use it a sense of control and can be practised in the course of ordinary daily living.

Michele, who learnt visualisation techniques at the Bristol Centre, applied them to her radiotherapy sessions. She said:

> ❝I visualised myself in special places and with healing light coming down, which was particularly helpful.❞

She added:

> ❝I wouldn't say I am incredibly well practised in visualisation – it's more about having hope and control ... there are all different sorts of therapies, but really all these things pulled together ... it's the philosophy of 'Your life really is in your hands'.❞

Reflexology

Reflexology is based on the theory that the feet mirror the body, and pressure areas (or reflex areas) on the feet correspond to all the different body organs and systems. The areas form a map of the body, with the right foot corresponding to the right side of the body and the left foot to the left side.

A reflexologist starts by taking a full medical history to indicate appropriate treatment. The therapist then applies gentle pressure with her thumbs to the various reflexes and interprets the patient's response to establish which parts of the body are functioning well and which are not. Reflexology is used to relieve tension and stress, to promote relaxation and boost the immune system. There is some evidence to support the claims of reflexologists to alleviate pain, but less to support their claims to diagnose effectively.

Alternative therapies

Alternative medical systems are complete structures of health theory and practice that are independent of conventional medicine. Many of them are thousands of years old and are still the preferred method of treatment in many cultures. Examples include traditional Chinese medicine, Ayurveda, homeopathic and naturopathic medicine.

Traditional Chinese medicine is based on the theory that the body's internal energy force (*qi*) regulates health and is kept in balance through various means such as a macrobiotic diet, Chinese herbal medicine, acupuncture, massage and meditation.

Ayurveda is the ancient system of the Indian continent, which suggests that disease is the result of an imbalance in the energies of the mind, body and forces of nature. It incorporates diet, herbal therapies, yoga, meditation, massage and imagery.

Laetrile, which is made from apricot stones, has been touted as a cure for cancer, but the Food and Drug Administration in America has prohibited its sale, with the warning that it has no known effect on cancer and breaks down in the body into highly toxic cyanide gas.

Practitioners of the Gerson diet, developed in the 1930s by Dr Max Gerson, from Germany, usually recommend it as an alternative to regular cancer treatment. They believe that cleansing the body of toxins will enable the body to recognise and kill cancer cells. In order to do this they use a special low-salt, high-potassium diet, nutritional supplements, coffee enemas and 20 lbs (9 kilos) of crushed fruit and vegetables each day to detoxify the body and strengthen the immune system. But there is no research to support their claims that their regime is successful in treating or curing cancer and the side effects of coffee enemas are potentially fatal. Nevertheless, the link between diet and cancer has been well established.

Diet and cancer

The role of nutrition in the development of cancer is increasingly coming under investigation. Cancer Research UK says the research suggests that between 10 and 70 per cent of cancers may be preventable by changing diet. But controlling people's diets in order to study by randomised controlled trials is not feasible. One alternative is to record the eating habits of a large group of healthy people over a period of time then follow them up to see who becomes ill and with what. A big, Europe-wide research project called EPIC (European Prospective Investigation into Cancer), which started in 1992, is doing just that and will report on diet and cancer over the next 10 to 20 years.

From a wide variety of studies so far, although the details differ, the evidence appears to be strong that a diet high in fruit, vegetables, pulses and whole foods, and low in fat, decreases the risk of cancer, while one high in red meat or meat that has been fried, animal fat, smoked and pickled foods and alcohol, increases it.

There has been a great deal of interest in the breast cancer rates of Japanese and American women. Japanese women living in Japan have a much lower rate of breast cancer than American women, but when they go to live in America their risk changes in line with their new neighbours. Researchers suspect that a soya-rich diet, high in phyto-oestrogens, reduces the risk of breast cancer, though not all studies bear this out and no conclusions can be made about the effect of soya on the risk of breast cancer or its effect on the course of breast cancer in women who already have it.

No anti-cancer diet has yet been shown to cure established cancers, but studies suggest that careful manipulation of the diet can improve the quality of life and actually prolong survival for some cancer patients. Unfortunately we cannot yet predict which cancers and which individuals will respond to specific dietary changes.

The most recent research points to the importance of plant chemicals known as phytochemicals, which might actually be able to boost the immune system, repair cellular damage and protect against dangerous genetic mutation.

But while we wait for a one-stop solution to cancer, there are things closer to the home and kitchen that will help. Foods such as broccoli, soya, oriental mushrooms, garlic and live yoghurt have been found to boost the immune system, block the effect of hormones on breast tissue, improve the liver's handling of carcinogens, and halt damage to DNA. Eating these foods might help to prevent breast cancer but will certainly, at worst, do no harm (see Box 7 for a summary).

Box 7. **Dietary recommendations.**

It could help to prevent breast cancer if you eat:

- Less saturated animal fat: replace with monounsaturated fat such as olive oil and polyunsaturated fats (vegetable oils and margarine).
- Less red meat or meat that has been fried.
- More poultry, fish and vegetable proteins such as beans, lentils or soya.
- More wheatbran fibre and wholemeal cereals.
- More fruit and vegetables, particularly those high in vitamin A.
- More starchy foods such as rice, pasta and potatoes.
- Less sugary processed foods such as cakes, biscuits and chocolate.
- Less alcohol.

Summary

- Complementary therapies are used alongside conventional medicine, while alternative therapies aim to replace it.

- Neither has been subjected to rigorous scientific scrutiny and their effectiveness is largely unproved.

- Most complementary therapies are not regulated by law, but they usually have a professional body and recognised qualifications to practise safely, which patients should check out before agreeing to treatment.

- The most commonly used for breast cancer are: acupuncture (and acupressure), aromatherapy, creative therapies, herbal medicine, homeopathy, hypnotherapy, relaxation and visualisation and reflexology.

- The Bristol Cancer Help Centre aims to provide a holistic approach and a place where 'body, mind and spirit could be thought about simultaneously' but under strong medical guidance.

- Alternative therapies such as laetrile and the Gerson diet make claims to cure cancer, but the sale of laetrile is illegal in the USA and the Gerson diet has no research to back up its claims.

- The evidence for the role of nutrition in developing cancer is increasingly convincing and, though no diet has been shown to cure cancer, studies suggest it can improve the quality of life and actually prolong survival for some patients.

Frequently asked questions

16

Does stress cause breast cancer?

Many scientific studies have looked at a possible link between stress and cancer, but there is no evidence that stress is a cause. Stressful events, such as bereavement, divorce and redundancy, are very common life events and it is more than likely that people with cancer will have experienced one or more within a few years' of their diagnosis. Doctors often don't know what caused the cancer and people usually seek their own explanation for it. Stress is something that seems feasible, but there is no scientific evidence to suggest that stressful events are any more common in the lives of cancer patients than the rest of the population. And no evidence that stress will precipitate a return of the disease. A study led by Professor Amanda Ramirez of Cancer Research UK's London Psychosocial Group (Graham *et al.*, 2002) found that 'women who have a severely stressful life experience in the year before being diagnosed with breast cancer, or in the five years afterwards, do not seem to be at increased risk' of it recurring.

Does abortion increase the risk of breast cancer?

A study funded by the pro-life/anti-abortion charity LIFE claimed that women who have an abortion face a higher risk of breast cancer. Their findings were based on a comparison of the numbers of women with breast cancer and the abortion rates in the UK, Finland, Sweden and the Czech Republic. They found that the increases in the two sets of figures matched and concluded that they were related. The Royal College of Obstetricians and Gynaecologists has examined the study, decided there is no causal link and accused LIFE of 'mischief making'.

Can antiperspirants cause breast cancer?

This seems to have arisen because of an email that was going the rounds suggesting that antiperspirant stops toxins being removed from the body in sweat so they build up in the lymph glands under the arm and cause breast cancer. Many women who are diagnosed with breast cancer have cancer cells in the lymph glands in the armpit, but the cancer originated in the breast, not in the lymph glands. A study reported in the *Journal of the National Cancer Institute* (Mirick *et al.*, 2002) found that there was no evidence that using deodorants or antiperspirants – either within an hour of shaving or not – increased the risk of developing breast cancer.

I am in my 30s and have already had surgery for four benign breast lumps – does this mean I am more likely to get breast cancer?

Benign breast lumps fall into two main groups: cysts that are filled with fluid; and those that are solid.

There is no evidence that breast cysts point to a higher risk of developing cancer. Solid lumps are more complicated. They can be divided into three types, depending on their appearance under a microscope: (1) non-proliferative; (2) proliferative; and (3) proliferative with atypia. There is no evidence that women with non-proliferative lumps are at higher risk of cancer. A woman who has a proliferative lump is about twice as likely to develop breast cancer during the following 20 years as a woman of the same age. A woman with the third type (proliferative with atypia) is around four or five times as likely to develop breast cancer as a woman of the same age who has not developed one. Doctors will always send solid benign breast lumps for microscopic examination and if there is any increased risk of cancer developing in the future they will suggest ways to keep an eye on the situation.

My 85-year-old mother has found a large lump in her breast and is refusing to see a doctor. Should I try to persuade her?

Breast cancer at this age usually progresses very slowly and even without treatment it could be several years before it caused any real problem. Once the cancer progresses, however, it could cause some very unpleasant and painful symptoms, or problems resulting from its spread to other parts of the body. The treatment for women with breast cancer at this age is often much less drastic than for younger women and might only involve taking medication such as tamoxifen, possibly combined with a relatively minor operation. Talking the situation over with a doctor might set your mother's mind at rest and in the end she would still have the right to refuse treatment.

Is it safe to eat soy if I'm on tamoxifen?

Soy first came under the spotlight when observational studies of women in different parts of the world revealed that women in Japan have much lower rates of breast cancer than in most European countries and the USA. One of the big differences is that the Japanese diet is high in soy. Soybeans, and many other plants like flaxseed, certain grains, beans, fruits, vegetables, and the roots ginseng and black cohosh contain natural plant chemicals called phyto-oestrogens (isoflavones) that mimic the female hormone oestrogen in the body. Some studies have found that eating phyto-oestrogens might give women without breast cancer some protection against developing it. But other studies have found no benefit and there is even some evidence that soy could be harmful. No one knows the answer, yet, and it is probably safer to keep consumption of soy protein down to one serving (40 grams) a day and to avoid capsule forms of soy, isoflavones or genestein if you have been diagnosed with breast cancer.

I am taking tamoxifen after surgery for breast cancer and now I am getting hot flushes. I have heard that red clover is helpful – is it safe for me to take?

Red clover contains isoflavonoids, which are very similar to the female hormone oestrogen, and could carry the same potential risks for women with breast cancer, so it would be wise to use with caution. Red clover also has the effect of thinning the blood, so is not suitable for anyone who is taking anticoagulant medication or has problems with abnormal bleeding.

I am 44 and have been treated for an early breast cancer. I have been told I will need regular mammograms but I am worried that I could get cancer because of the radiation – are these check-ups necessary, and are they safe?

National guidelines recommend a mammogram at least every two years after treatment for early breast cancer to check that there is no sign of recurrence or a new cancer. Mammograms do deliver a small dose of radiation to the breasts and there is a very small risk that this could cause a cancer to develop. The risk has been estimated at one extra cancer for every 100 000 women attending for routine mammography. The risk of developing breast cancer is greater in women who have previously been diagnosed than in the general population, so mammography gives a worthwhile benefit of early detection.

I had a lumpectomy and radiotherapy three years ago, but I have discovered another lump in the same breast. What treatment can I have?

Your doctor will usually recommend a mastectomy if the original cancer returns or a new one develops in the same breast. This is because further cancerous changes are likely and removing the lump would not solve the problem, also you could not have any further radiotherapy on that breast.

I have an identical twin sister who has breast cancer – what is my risk?

Recent research suggests that identical twins of women who have already been diagnosed with breast cancer are three to four times more likely to develop the disease than the average woman. Identical twin sisters are genetically the same and the genetic component is an important contributory factor in breast cancer, though environmental factors are also involved. The BRCA1 and BRCA2 genes are known greatly to increase the risk of breast cancer, but they only account for about 2 per cent of all breast cancers. It is believed that inherited risk is probably more often caused by the interaction of a number of different genes with the environment.

Glossary

Adenocarcinoma   A cancer that arises in gland-forming tissue. Breast cancer is a type of adenocarcinoma.

Adjuvant therapy   Treatment that is given in addition to the primary treatment, to enhance its effectiveness. Surgery is the usual primary treatment for breast cancer, while chemotherapy, radiotherapy and hormone treatments are often given additionally.

Advanced (metastatic) breast cancer   Breast cancer that has spread from the breast to other parts of the body, through the bloodstream or lymph system.

Alopoecia   Hair loss, a common side effect of chemotherapy.

Apoptosis   Cell suicide.

Aspiration   Putting a hypodermic needle into tissue and drawing back on the syringe to remove fluid or cells.

Atypical cell   A cell which is mildly to moderately abnormal.

Atypical hyperplasia   Cells that are not only growing abnormally but have increased in number.

Axilla   Armpit.

Axillary lymph nodes   Lymph nodes found in the armpit.

Axillary lymph node dissection   Surgical removal of the lymph nodes from the armpit.

Benign   Not cancerous. This means it cannot invade other parts of the body.

Bilateral   Involving both sides, such as both breasts.

Biopsy   Removal of tissue, but this does not indicate how much tissue will be removed.

Bone scan   A test to determine if there is any sign of cancer in the bones.

Breast reconstruction   Creation of an artificial breast after mastectomy.

Calcification   Small calcium deposits in tissue which can be seen by mammography. They are often associated with benign changes, but can indicate cancer.

Carcinogen   Substance that can cause cancer.

Carcinoma   Cancer that arises from epithelial tissues (skin, glands and lining of internal organs). The majority of cancers are carcinomas.

Cell cycle   The stages a cell goes through to reproduce itself.

Carcinoma in situ   Cancer cells are present, but are confined to the area where they started and have not yet spread to surrounding tissues, which means they have not spread to other parts of the body.

Chemotherapy   The use of certain chemicals to treat disease. The term usually refers to cytotoxic drugs used to treat cancer.

Core biopsy   A type of needle biopsy, where a small core of tissue is removed from a tumour without surgery.

Cyst   Fluid-filled sac. Breast cysts are benign.

Cytology   The study of cells.

Cytotoxic   Poisonous to cells. The term usually refers to drugs used in chemotherapy.

Diethylstilbestrol (DES)   Synthetic oestrogen once used to prevent miscarriages and stop milk production, now known to cause vaginal cancer in the daughters of the women who took it and sometimes used to treat metastatic breast cancer.

Ductal carcinoma in situ (DCIS)   Ductal cancer cells that have not grown out of the ducts of the breast tissue where they originated. Sometimes referred to as pre-cancerous.

Excisional biopsy   The whole lump is removed.

Fibroadenoma   Non-cancerous fibrous lump in the breast most commonly found in young women.

Follicle stimulating hormone (FSH)   Hormone from the pituitary gland used to stimulate the ovary to produce eggs.

Haemotoma   Collection of blood in the tissues which can happen in the breast after surgery.

Hormones   Chemical substances produced by glands in the body which enter the bloodstream and affect organs and tissues throughout the body.

Hot flushes   Sudden sensations of heat and swelling associated with the menopause and side effects of hormonal therapies such as tamoxifen.

Hyperplasia   Excessive growth of cells.

Incisional biopsy   A portion of the tumour is removed for diagnosis.

In situ   In its original site. In cancer, this refers to tumours that have not spread beyond their original site and invaded neighbouring tissues.

Invasive cancer   Cancer that is capable of spreading into nearby tissue; but this does not imply it is aggressive or has already spread outside the breast.

Latissimus flap   Flap of skin and muscle taken from the back and used for breast reconstruction.

Lobules   Parts of the breast capable of making milk.

Local recurrence   Cancer which returns in the original tumour site.

Lumpectomy   Surgery to remove only the breast lump and a small surrounding area of normal tissue.

Lymph nodes   Glands throughout the body which help defend against bacteria. They can indicate whether the cancer has spread to the rest of the body.

Lymphoedema   Swelling of the arm that can happen following surgery to the lymph nodes in the armpit. It can happen immediately or years later and can be temporary or permanent.

Malignant   Cancerous – tumours that can invade neighbouring tissues or spread to other parts of the body.

Mammogram   An X-ray of the breast.

Mastectomy   Surgery to remove the breast tissue, or as much of it as possible.

Metastasis   Spread of cancer to another organ, through the bloodstream or lymph system. Metastasised tumours are ones that have spread to other parts of the body, but whose cancer cells are the same as those in the place of origin (the primary tumour).

Neoadjuvant therapy   A treatment that is given in addition to the primary therapy but before it. If chemotherapy is given before surgery it is called neoadjuvant.

Oncology   The study of cancer.

Oophorectomy   Removal of the ovaries.

Palliation   Relieving the symptom, without curing the disease.

Palpation   A technique in which the doctor presses on the body's surface to feel the organs or tissues beneath.

Pathologist   A specialist who identifies diseases by studying cells and tissues under a microscope.

Prophylactic   Preventative medicine.

Prognosis   Expected or likely outcome.

Prosthesis   An artificial replacement for a part of the body, as in breast prosthesis.

Radiation therapy   Treatment with high-energy rays (such as X-rays) to kill cancer cells.

Randomised controlled study   A study in which the participants are chosen at random to receive a particular treatment.

Recurrence   Return of cancer after it had apparently completely disappeared.

Remission   Disappearance of any detectable disease.

SERM   Selective oestrogen receptor modulator: a compound which is oestrogenic in some organs and anti-oestrogenic in others.

Seroma   Collection of tissue fluid.

Systemic treatment   Treatment that involves the whole body, usually using drugs.

Tumour   An abnormal mass of tissue, which can be either benign or cancerous.

Useful addresses and contacts

General

Breast Cancer Care

Breast Cancer Care is the main organisation in the UK providing information and support for anyone affected by breast cancer. Its services are free and include a helpline, website, publications and practical and emotional support.

Address: Kiln House
                    210 New Kings Road
                    London SW6 4NZ
Telephone: Helpline 0808 800 6000 Mon–Fri 10am–5pm
Email: info@breastcancercare.org.uk
Web address: www.breastcancer.org.uk

Cancer BACUP

This provides a major cancer information service along with practical advice and support for cancer patients, their families and carers.

Address: 3 Bath Place
                    Rivington Street
                    London EC2A 3JR
Telephone: Helpline 0808 800 1234 Mon–Fri 9am–7pm
                    Switchboard 020 7696 9003 Mon–Fri 9am–5.30pm
Web address: www.cancerbacup.org.uk

Cancer Research UK

Cancer Research UK is a UK research charity which undertakes world-class scientific research into the biology and causes of cancer, with a view to developing effective treatments. It is also an excellent source of authoritative information on all the different types of cancer.

Address: PO Box 123
                    Lincoln's Inn Fields
                    London WC2A 3PX
Telephone: Customer services 020 7009 8820
                    Switchboard 020 7242 0200
Web address: www.cancerresearchuk.org

Macmillan Cancer Relief

This is a UK charity that works to improve the quality of life for people living with cancer. Macmillan nurses advise patients on the different treatments and support them and their families throughout the illness from the point of diagnosis. They don't provide basic practical nursing care within the home or domestic help.

Address:	89 Albert Embankment
	London SE1 7YQ
Telephone:	Helpline 0808 808 2020 Mon–Fri 9am–6pm
	Textphone 0808 808 0121
	Switchboard 020 7840 7840
Email:	cancerline@macmillan.org.uk
Web address:	www.macmillan.org.uk

Marie Curie Cancer Care

Marie Curie nurses provide free care in the community for cancer patients who are terminally ill, giving them the chance to die at home, supported by their families. There are also ten Marie Curie hospices.

Address:	89 Albert Embankment
	London SE1 7TP
Telephone:	020 7599 7777
Web address:	www.mariecurie.org.uk

NHS Direct

This is a confidential telephone advice line staffed by nurses, open 24 hours a day, 365 days of the year. There is also an internet-based NHS direct service.

Telephone:	0845 4647
Web address:	www.nhsdirect.nhs.uk

UK Breast Cancer Coalition

This was founded in 1995 by women with personal experience of breast cancer. It aims to increase patients' influence in treatment decisions.

Address:	1D Broadway House
	112–134 The Broadway
	Wimbledon SW19 1RL
Telephone:	020 8543 4455
Email:	info@ukbcc.org.uk
Web address:	www.ukbcc.org.uk

Psychological help

British Psychological Society

This is the representative body for psychologists in the UK. It has a register of chartered psychologists, where members of the public can search for a suitably qualified professional.

Address:	St Andrews House
	48 Princess Road East
	Leicester LE1 7DR
Telephone:	0116 254 9568
Email:	enquiry@bps.org.uk
Web address:	www.bps.org.uk

Complementary therapies

The Bristol Cancer Help Centre

This is the UK's leading holistic cancer charity for people with cancer and those close to them. The Bristol Approach, pioneered by the charity, works alongside medical treatment, offering a combination of physical, emotional and spiritual support, using complementary therapies and self-help techniques in 2- or 5-day residential courses.

Address:	Grove House
	Cornwallis Grove
	Bristol BS8 4PG
Telephone:	Helpline 0845 123 2310
Email:	helpline@bristolcancerhelp.org
Web address:	www.bristolcancerhelp.org

The British Medical Acupuncture Society

The BMAS is a registered charity set up to encourage the use and scientific understanding of acupuncture within medicine for the public benefit. It was formed in 1980 as an association of medical practitioners interested in acupuncture and there are now more than 2300 members who use acupuncture in hospital or general practice. A list of practitioners is available from the office or on the website.

Address:	The Administrator, BMAS
	3 Winnington Court
	Northwich CW8 1AQ

Telephone: 01606 786782
Email: Admin@medical-acupuncture.org.uk
Web address: www.medical-acupuncture.co.uk

The Research Council for Complementary Medicine

The RCCM, founded in 1983 by practitioners and researchers from both orthodox and complementary medicine, aims to develop and extend the evidence base for complementary medicine and to provide information about the effectiveness of therapies and treatment for specific conditions. It does not recommend any specific treatment option.

Address: 27a Devonshire Street
                    London W1G 6PN
Telephone: 020 7935 7499
Email: info@rccm.org.uk
Web address: www.rccm.org.uk

Register of Chinese Herbal Medicine

This was set up in 1987 to regulate the practice of Chinese herbal medicine in the UK and will provide a list of qualified practitioners.

Address: Office 5
                    1 Exeter Street
                    Norwich NR2 4QB
Telephone: 01603 623994
Email: herbmed@rchm.co.uk
Web address: www.rchm.co.uk

Other helpful organisations

Lymphoedema Support Network

This is a registered national charity, founded in 1991 by a group of people with lymphoedema. It provides information and support to people with lymphoedema, with a telephone helpline, quarterly newsletter and wide range of fact sheets, a website and self-help videos.

Address: St Luke's Crypt
                    Sydney Street
                    London SW3 6NH

Telephone: Information and support 020 7351 4480
                Administration 020 7351 0990
Web address: www.lymphoedema.org

An Arm and a Leg Limited

This offers a 20-day residential treatment for lymphoedema, involving Decongestive Lymphatic Therapy which includes twice daily manual lymph drainage and multilayer lymphoedema bandaging, combined with physiotherapy and aquatherapy.

Address: PO Box 22920
                London N10 3WU
Telephone: 07071 229865
Email: info@anarmandaleg.co.uk
Web address: www.anarmandaleg.co.uk

Amoena (UK) Ltd

These are makers and retailers of breast prostheses (including an adhesive breast form), prosthetic nipples, mastectomy lingerie and swimwear.

Address: FREEPOST
                Eastleigh
                Hampshire SO53 4BJ
Telephone: 0800 072 6636 Mon–Fri 9am–5pm
Web address: www.amoena.co.uk

Nicola Jane

A company that produces a specialist range of bras and swimwear for use after breast surgery.

Telephone: 01243 533188
Email: info@nicolajane.com
Web address: www.nicolajane.com

Hair Development (UK) Ltd

This is a wig supplier, offering specialist advice after hair loss from chemotherapy.

Telephone: 020 7790 3996
Email: hair@hair-development.com
Web address: www.hair-development.com

Headline Hats

This company supplies an attractive alternative to wigs for people with hair loss.

Telephone: 020 8874 1099
Email: sales@headlinehats.co.uk
Web address: www.headlinehats.co.uk

References

Bernstein, L., Deapen, D., Cerhan, J.R., Schwartz, S.M., Liff, J., McGann-Maloney, E., Perlman, J.A. & Ford, L. (1999). Tamoxifen therapy for breast cancer and endometrial cancer risk. *Journal of the National Cancer Institute*, **91**(19), 1654–62.

Brown, Z. & Leffall, L.D. (2003). *100 Questions and Answers About Breast Cancer.* Sudbury, MA: Jones and Bartlett Publishers.

Cancer Research UK (2002). *Breast Cancer: Spot the Symptoms Early* (Leaflet). London: Cancer Research UK.

Cuzick, J., Powles, T., Veronesi, U., Forbes, J., Edwards, R., Ashley, S. & Boyle, P. (2003). Overview of the main outcomes in breast cancer prevention trials. *The Lancet*, **361**, 296–300.

Graham, J., Ramirez, A., Love, S., Richards, M. & Burgess, C. (2002). Stressful life experiences and risk of relapse of breast cancer: Observational cohort study. *British Medical Journal*, **324**, 1420–22.

Iredale, R. (2003) Breast cancer in men: Group is exploring issues for men with breast cancer across the United Kingdom. *British Medical Journal*, **327**, 930–1 (18 October). The MATCH project (men's attitudes towards cancer and health), Rachel Iredale, senior research fellow, Institute of Medical Genetics, University of Wales College of Medicine, Cardiff.

Kaufmann, M., Jonat, W., Blamey, R., Cuzick, J., Namer, M., Fogelman, I., de Haes, J.C., Schumacher, M. & Sauerbrei, W. (Zoladex Early Breast Cancer Research Association (ZEBRA) Trialists' Group) (2003). Survival analyses from the ZEBRA study: Goserelin (Zoladex) versus CMF in premenopausal women with node-positive breast cancer. *European Journal of Cancer*, **39**(12), 1711–17.

Mirick, D.K., Davis, S., Thomas, D.B. (2002). Antiperspirant use and the risk of breast cancer. *Journal of the National Cancer Institute*, **94**(20), 1578–80.

NHS Cancer Screening Programmes website: www.cancerscreening.nhs.uk.

Index

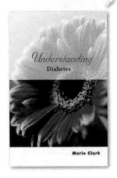
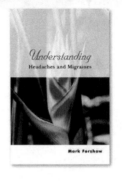